Doctor Robert Lefever

The Promis Recovery Centre

dangerous doctors

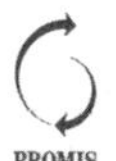

Written by Dr Robert Lefever

PROMIS Recovery Centre Limited
The Old Court House, Pinners Hill
Nonington, Nr. Canterbury
Kent CT15 4LL. UK
www.promis.co.uk

ISBN 1 871013 17 8

Design and production by Rainbow, Ipswich IP5 3RY, England.
Printed in Basauri, Spain by Grafo SA.

To
my friends and patients
Jeffrey and Aline Robinson
and their children Joshua and Seline

Acknowledgements

To my secretary, Sarah Oaten, for typing the manuscript

To my editor, Dr Harriet Harvey Wood, for her encouragement and exceedingly helpful suggestions.

To my proof reader, Keith Burns, for going beyond the line of duty.

To my patients for their forbearance.

Contents

“To know and yet think we do not know is the highest attainment.
Not to know and yet think we do is a disease.”

Lao-tzu.

Chapter One

Mistakes

To the challenge that I am undermining people's faith in their doctors, I would reply that I should hope so: doctors should rely upon professionalism rather than upon blind faith.

To the challenge from the dean of a medical school that I unsettled students in their convictions, I replied that I was glad of that: students should learn to think for themselves and be excited by discovering new ideas; they should learn to work things out for themselves as well as learning basic disciplined thought processes; they should learn to look things up or ask other people for help rather than rely upon imperfect memory.

Medical school training has a lot to answer for. As Professor Lawrence Weed of the University of Vermont points out (*Medical Records, Medical Education and Patient Care*, Yearbook Publications 1969), it tends to prepare students for examinations in which the basic question is "What do you know?" rather than "How would you work it out?" or "How would you react when you don't know?". In clinical practice as working doctors we mostly have to make decisions on inadequate information. The only doctors who can see near enough the full truth of a patient's condition are post-mortem pathologists. Those of us who work with patients who are still alive have to make our best guess at some stage, or even several stages, in every consultation.

It is inevitable that when we guess we sometimes make mistakes. The art of clinical practice is not only to cut down our mistakes by examining patients thoroughly, doing appropriate clinical investigations – and then making proper records so that other doctors can follow us responsibly – but also to do all these things in the real world where there are administrative, practical, temporal and financial constraints.

Yet even then, after bearing all these things in mind, we make mistakes – some of them idiotic. We have computers to guide us and help our memories. Some of us use Problem/Knowledge Coupler software to inform or remind us of diagnoses we may have overlooked. Yet still we make mistakes. In part this is inevitable. In the course of my professional life as a general medical practitioner I have done over a quarter of a million consultations. In some I made glaring errors which I have found out later when informed of them by the patient or another doctor or even by my wife who works with me partly as a physiotherapist and family counsellor but, as with the personal partners of many doctors, more as my "minder" – challenging me as much as supporting me. Also I am sure that I make many mistakes that never come to light. In the last analysis I am sure that I make some form of error of commission or omission in every consultation. I do not ask for understanding on "human error". I simply make the point that perfection is impossible.

Sometimes, when I read reports from the Medical Protection Society, or in the newspapers when they give accounts of hearings of the General Medical Council, I think to myself that the errant doctor deserved his or her fate. At other times I have a shudder of fear in knowing that any one of us could have been caught out on that particular issue. Health Authorities, the courts and the press occasionally have a "red hot" issue of the moment and one can almost guarantee that some doctor somewhere will be singled out for professional vilification as a warning to the rest of us. That is unfair.

It seems to me, however, that the greatest problems are cultural rather than individual. It is fair enough when an individual doctor is blamed for a mistake, give or take whether the error was understandable or crass. It is altogether another matter when an entire profession is criticised cynically in "shock ... horror" articles, books, lectures or Government reports. The particular feature that concerns me is that these challenges might sometimes be justified yet still have the opposite effect to that which was intended. Far from leading to improvements in standards, the constant harassment of the medical profession is just as damaging at one extreme as constant deification would be at the other. We have to examine the whole culture of our medical and legal systems and the role of pressure groups, public bodies, Parliament and the press. We get the medical profession we deserve. If society makes doctors defensive, through The National Patient Safety Agency, we will behave defensively. If society has unreasonable expectations, we will be *more* likely to make mistakes.

That being said, there are times – perhaps particularly in the field of mental illness – when the medical profession has become arrogant and blind to the true needs of the population we serve. As the Los Angeles psychiatrist and creator of *Choice Theory* (Harper Perennial 1998), Dr William Glasser, points out, "When someone says 'I know what's good for you', we should run for our lives".

Being a doctor is one of the greatest privileges on earth. The scientific and human challenges are immense and therefore potentially incredibly rewarding or destructive. Ultimately each doctor, like anyone else, is responsible for his or her own thoughts, feelings, actions and reactions. We cannot hand on the responsibility for any of these individual characteristics to anyone else. It is simply untrue to say "I had to ..." or "They made me ..." or any other statement that implies that we are mere robots. Nevertheless, the sense of personal responsibility is easily lost when doctors come to feel victimised in their work.

Blaming doctors is easy. Blaming ourselves in our work as doctors is also easy, distressingly so at times. We, as much as other people, may have superhuman expectations of ourselves. The crucial issue is not to see whether we make mistakes – of course we do – but why we make them. In this it is the doctor's internal psychological processes that are perhaps the greatest influence: those who have lost their enthusiasm will inevitably do bad work. Seeing what doctors do wrong is therefore only the start – and the easy bit at that. It is more important to consider how and why we get to the psychological state in which we are more likely to make mistakes.

A GP friend of mine, who has spent his entire professional life caring for patients in the National Health Service said to me recently "I don't enjoy my work any more. I just do it". That is a tragedy – and a dangerous one.

Chapter Two

Physical Harm

There is a particular level of trust that we place in our doctors. We trust other professionals such as our lawyers, accountants and architects, and their inevitable occasional mistakes can cause inconvenience, sometimes considerably so. The mistakes of doctors can cause a lot more than that. Medical procedures or surgical operations can relieve or cure but they can also damage or even kill. In the security of our homes we can search the Internet for medical information but it can never give us clinical judgement: for that we have to trust our doctors. Furthermore, when we submit ourselves to the care of doctors, we may be frightened or in pain and therefore least able to make a rational judgement for ourselves. Under general anaesthetic we are totally powerless.

We trust our doctors because we have to. That is why it is so particularly disturbing when doctors make mistakes or when, in other ways, they show themselves to be unworthy of our trust. We believe anything rather than that. I remember visiting Budapest when it was under Communist rule. In a hospital Accident and Emergency Department I saw mud and blood on the floor. My guide explained, "We have poor facilities but our doctors are wonderful". Manifestly that was untrue: any responsible doctor would have concentrated first of all on reducing the risk of sepsis. However, I could not say that to my guide: she had to believe in her doctors because she had no alternative.

This is an extremely important point. When we consider the philosophical, political, financial, administrative and clinical principles of a health service, wherever in the world we may be, we may find it extremely difficult to consider the issues in broad terms rather than in the parochial terms of our own country's health and welfare system. For example, the British National Health Service has been repeatedly claimed by some of our own politicians to be "the envy of the world". The fact that no other country has copied it is simply ignored. Such failings as may have been acknowledged are usually put down to inadequate funding, poor administration or avaricious doctors who spend too much of their time and attention on their private fee-paying patients. It rarely occurs to anyone to challenge the basic philosophical and political principles upon which the NHS is based. However, this is exactly what we must do if we are to see where and why things go wrong despite repeated reorganisations of the system and despite recent massive injections of financial capital.

Pointing out the deficiencies in the healthcare system does not excuse doctors for our individual mistakes. However (and I speak as one who has not worked in the NHS since 1980) I do believe that the working conditions of doctors in the NHS make it more likely that they will make mistakes than if they were to work in the private sector. Obviously there are significant clinical, financial, administrative and other factors that need to be taken into account in the particular working conditions of each doctor. Nonetheless I stick to my basic point that doctors and other healthcare workers are less likely to make mistakes when they feel happy and fulfilled in their clinical environment and in the work that they do. When their hearts and minds are at peace, and they are less preoccupied, it is obvious that they will be better able to focus their attention on the clinical care of their patients.

Some doctors, particularly those who are drunk or drug-addicted (doctors get the same problems as anyone else), are more likely to make mistakes than others. Similarly, doctors who are preoccupied with personal issues such as divorce or other family tragedies will also have their minds distracted by these personal worries. Doctors who are too tired because they are too busy, will be particularly at risk of making mistakes. Doctors whose attention is primarily focused upon their own professional advancement may lose sight of some of the basic human rights of their patients and may make poor judgement on what is or is not necessary and helpful. Doctors whose minds are targeted more upon their own perceived entitlements than upon the care of their patients will become instruments of harm rather than help. Doctors who are not enjoying their work and who do not look forward to each new day, will soon become de-skilled and slide gradually and inexorably towards incompetence.

I believe that it is for these reasons that doctors sometimes make mistakes, which should be totally avoidable. Consider the following examples:

Avoidable Mistakes

The wrong patient

Sometimes there is a failure to check the identity of the patient. This is obviously most important with patients who are unconscious as a result of anaesthesia prior to surgery. However, it can happen at any time, particularly if the doctor picks up the wrong set of medical records. Sometimes there is confusion when patients have similar or even identical names. Names such as Amin, Patel, or Singh are particularly common because they refer more to tribal or religious groups than family origin, yet even some typically English names – such as John Smith – can be dangerously common. I recall one medico-legal case where two patients on the same ward had the same name but the first name and surname were the other way round – as in Paul John and John Paul. That is extraordinarily bad luck both for the patients and for the doctor – but it is exactly this type of issue that becomes a problem when doctors are tired or preoccupied. The most common problem of this nature, however, most probably occurs when the doctor has two sets of notes on his or her desk and writes the wrong name on the pathology sample or other clinical investigation. It is easy for doctors who are overworked and overtired to make this type of mistake.

The wrong operation

This is sometimes done on the wrong patient altogether when the wrong records are supplied with an unconscious patient but, more commonly, the operation is done on the correct patient but on the wrong side of the body. Considering the sheer number of operations that are done, it is almost inevitable that a mistake of this kind will happen every so often. The truly remarkable feature is the vast number of operations that are carried out successfully. It is nonetheless indefensible when this type of error occurs and one has to consider all the individual and clinical factors involved when such totally unacceptable mistakes occur. Were some individual personalities destructive rather than co-operative within the surgical team? Was morale generally depressed within that department or hospital because of economic, administrative or general political issues?

Anaesthetic accidents

Sometimes there is a blocked tube or the gas bottle runs out, or the wrong gas or other drug is given, or the drug was given by the wrong route such as intravenous rather than intramuscular. All these things can happen and it is for this reason that doctors themselves, when they are patients, take care to find out as much about the anaesthetist as about the surgeon. It was said that Lord Nuffield, when he endowed a professorship of Anaesthesia at Oxford University as well as professorships of Medicine, Surgery and Obstetrics and Gynaecology, replied to the statement that "Any fool could give an anaesthetic" with the withering response "That was exactly my fear".

The wrong medicine

Some drugs have similar names and a simple confusion may occur. On other occasions the doctor may give the wrong drug for a particular condition. More commonly the right drug is given but in the wrong dose. Decimal points in the wrong place can be a particular problem for infants when they may be given 10 or even 100 times the appropriate dose.

The wrong site

Drugs can be given through the skin (transdermal), into the skin (intradermal), under the skin (subcutaneous), into the muscles (intramuscular), into the veins (intravenous) or into the spinal canal (intrathecal). Disasters occur on occasions when the right drug is given but into the wrong place. Again it is pointless to ask, "How could this possibly happen?". The fact is that it does happen and one needs to ask, "What pressures was the doctor under?". Sometimes good doctors do bad things. Obviously we should be concerned that bad doctors should be weeded out and prevented from making repeated errors. However, if good doctors are prevented from continuing in clinical practice after making any significant error, then there would be very few doctors left in clinical practice.

Possibly Avoidable Mistakes

The next group of mistakes are those that are possibly avoidable but more understandable when they occur.

Drug interactions

There is a vast amount of data on potential drug interactions. Much of this is nowadays computerised so that warnings are flashed up on the screen to remind doctors of potential pitfalls. Even so, mistakes can happen. The courts sometimes have totally unreasonable expectations in requiring doctors to inform patients of every possible side effect and to record in their notes that they have done so. This is a prime example of the occasions when any doctor could get caught out. It is a totally unrealistic expectation and has no insight whatever into time constraints or any of the other simple practicalities of clinical life.

Drug side effects

As with drug interactions, a vast amount is known - and much of this is computerised - yet errors are difficult to avoid. One may be aware of potential side effects but there is usually no way of knowing whether a particular patient will develop one or another side effect. Some people die of an acute allergic reaction following one tablet of aspirin or penicillin. This idiosyncratic response is a disaster for the individual patient and a sad occurrence for the individual doctor, but it does not mean that we should all stop prescribing aspirin or penicillin or other drugs that may have these idiosyncratic allergic responses. Some people may have excessive responses to certain substances, e.g. an allergy to nuts or bee-stings, but one may never find this out until after the event. The courts are generally understanding of this problem but they can still be unreasonable in their expectation that doctors should warn patients of all possible side effects of drugs and record in their notes that they have done so.

Making the wrong diagnosis

Doctors are trained to follow basic clinical disciplines and nowadays the use of Problem Knowledge Couplers (in which the computer stores up-to-date knowledge on a subject and the doctor puts in the clinical data from the patient in order to obtain appropriate reminders) or other computer-assisted diagnostic and therapeutic tools can reduce the level of risk, particularly when we acknowledge that human memory is fallible. However, computers can never provide judgement: only human beings can do that - and all judgements are fallible. Even the top super-specialists in the world make mistakes in their own field of expertise, let alone in other areas. GPs have absolutely no chance of knowing everything about everything. The most that can be asked of any of us is that our medical records should reveal our observations and thought processes.

Missing the diagnosis altogether

Some diseases - such as thyroid deficiency - come on gradually and a doctor who knows the patient well may not see this gradual change whereas a new doctor, seeing the patient for the first time, will recognise the condition immediately. This is a classic error that all medical students are taught to avoid. Nonetheless, inevitably, it still happens. A more common cause of missing a diagnosis is that the doctor did not listen accurately to the patient's description of his or her symptoms, or did not examine him or her properly or do the right tests or make the right referrals for further opinion. Sometimes doctors may be out of date or simply lazy or preoccupied or dispirited. This can happen at any age and is not simply a problem associated with older doctors. Similarly, doctors can be ignorant or isolated even when working alongside a group of other doctors. Single-handed practice can be an inspiration rather than a handicap in general medical practice. In general, the doctor's prime responsibility must surely be to be good at what he or she sees most commonly and then to recognise that help is needed when rare conditions turn up. Both undergraduate and postgraduate education sometimes completely miss this point. General medical practitioners are often trained by hospital doctors who have particular interests in subjects that GPs may rarely see in clinical practice.

For example, I was trained extensively in the diagnosis of rheumatic fever and rheumatic heart disease but have seen only one case of acute rheumatic fever in my entire professional life. I therefore really do not need to know a great deal about acute rheumatic fever – only that it exists and that I need to refer the patient on to a specialist if I do ever come across a case. Furthermore, I would consider it perfectly appropriate for a patient who suffers from rheumatic fever to know more about it than I do. I have a responsibility to know more than he or she does on a vast number of other subjects. Patients are sometimes upset by this attitude. They may expect me, as their own personal general medical practitioner, to be so interested in their particular condition that I should spend the small hours surfing the Internet for every possible piece of information on their particular problem.

As in all things, doctors have to make judgements on what we can reasonably be expected to know and what we should delegate to others. In general medical practice we inevitably become relatively expert in the things that we see frequently and relatively ignorant on the things that we do not see. For example, I work in South Kensington in central London and look after a young population in "bed-sit" land. I have seen only one heart attack in the last twenty years. I have only one patient in a wheelchair. If I were to work in a south coast "retirement" area, my experience might well be almost the opposite. Thus it is unreasonable to expect all doctors to be expert in all things. Equally it is no solution to the problem to get large numbers of doctors to work together in massive group practices. That risks losing the personal touch that to my mind is the essence of general medical practice.

Poor judgement

Doctors may have an immense amount of helpful data available to them from a wide range of sources and yet still make poor judgement. Some are slapdash and always were, some are worn out physically and some are worn out emotionally.

Professor Lawrence Weed of the University of Vermont, in looking at this problem, believes that there are four behavioural constants:

i. Efficiency: doing things in as straightforward a manner as possible.
ii. Reliability: doing what one says one will do.
iii. Thoroughness: doing each part effectively.
iv. Analytical sense: making sensible conclusions when observing the data.

The important observation by Professor Weed is that each of us tends to be constant in these respects. For example, we may tend always to have a good analytical sense but nonetheless be unreliable. Professor Weed's recommendation is that doctors should be aware of our individual assets and liabilities in these behavioural constants and should make allowances for them. If we tend to be inefficient or unreliable, then we need to know that and use other staff to monitor us. It is not sufficient simply to try to buck ourselves up. We will not be able to do that – precisely because we tend to be inefficient or unreliable. Correspondingly, if we have a poor analytical sense then we will be in danger of causing a lot of damage to our patients and we would need to follow strict protocols for our clinical behaviour and refer on to other doctors immediately we are out of our depth.

Being out of our depth is not as rare, nor as dangerous nor as humiliating, as might at first appear. For example, I pride myself on my knowledge of addiction because that is a special interest of mine but I do not pride myself on my neurological knowledge. Neurology is an exceedingly complex subject and I have no hesitation in immediately referring to a consultant specialist any patient with a neurological problem. There is no shame in acknowledging when I don't know something: it would be stupid and dangerous to pretend otherwise.

Giving the wrong treatment

Obviously we sometimes make mistakes: the more simple the mistake, the more commonly it will occur. Prescribing a drug to which the patient is known to be allergic is a common error when doctors forget to ask the all-important question or fail to look at our notes for information we already possess. Another common error comes as a result of simple misdiagnosis. A doctor may prescribe exactly the right treatment for a particular condition – but the patient actually had something else. For example, an inflamed lump might be thought to be an abscess, for which the correct treatment would be an antibiotic, but it might in fact be due to a malignancy. That particular error can, with luck, be corrected very quickly when the inflammation does not respond after a week. However, there are times when doctors get stuck in diagnostic ruts so that we see what we believe we see. Continuing postgraduate education is obviously helpful in reminding us of wider possibilities but, even so, some doctors get diagnostic bees in their bonnets and repeatedly see things that the rest of us would not see in the same frequency or even at all. For example, the diagnosis food allergies is a contentious issues: some doctors believe that they are common and therefore diagnose them frequently. Others do not. Similarly, post-viral syndrome (myalgic encephalopathy or M.E.) does occur, but for some doctors it would be a daily diagnosis whereas others would acknowledge its existence much less commonly and would be more likely to make an emotional diagnosis on many of the patients who claim to have M.E..

Wrong data

Mention has already been made of the possibility of putting the wrong name on a pathological sample. A more common error comes as a result of trusting a test result when it simply does not fit with the patient's general medical condition. The sensible thing to do is to repeat the test or to telephone the specialist to ask him or her to look again.Significant errors can occur when doctors treat the false test result rather than the patient who was manifestly well.

Professional Errors

The next group of errors are those that could be described as "professional" errors. These relate to the way in which we run our medical practice rather than anything to do with clinical conditions as such. Nonetheless, the end results can be just as devastating to our patients.

Poor medical records

No doctor can provide 24-hour care for 365 days a year. Good medical records are therefore the instruments of continuing care and supervision for our patients. Problem-oriented medical records should be a basic discipline for all doctors. In these the subjective statements of the patient are recorded separately from the objective findings of the doctor. The clinical assessment is then recorded and plans are made for further investigation or treatment. The educational comments made to the patient on his or her condition are noted and the recommended therapeutic processes or medications are also recorded. The separation of all medical records into these component parts enables other doctors to distinguish between what was fact and what was the opinion of the doctor making the record. In this way the bad records of a good doctor have no value to anyone else whereas the good records of a bad doctor can at least reveal the diagnostic and therapeutic errors while at the same time providing valuable information on the actual concerns of the patient and some specific clinical findings.

Computerisation is a mixed blessing. It is commonplace to note that if one puts garbage into a computer file, one gets garbage out. There is little point in computerising records that are not already problem-oriented. In my view, Professor Weed's Problem Oriented Medical Information System (PROMIS) is an essential prerequisite for computerisation of medical records. Only by structuring the data in advance can one use a computer for appropriate cross-referencing and counting – the things it does best. A great deal of current computerisation of medical records achieves no more than could be done with a typewriter or photocopier or even a fountain pen and a telephone or fax machine. We fool ourselves if we believe that computerisation takes away the need for disciplined thought processes or that it necessarily supersedes more simple, straightforward approaches.

In the UK National Health Service the computerisation of medical data can be used sensibly in screening large populations and noting demographic data that can then be useful in determining appropriate policies concerning care for large populations. However, in the microcosm of an individual clinical practice, there is a great deal more to be done than simply monitoring chronic illnesses and recording inoculations, cervical smear tests and drug prescriptions in order to provide data for the Department of Health. All these recordings have their place and computers are indeed the appropriate tools for monitoring what has been done and therefore what has not been done. However, there is still a fundamental place for care and compassion in clinical practice – and these cannot be computerised. Of course there is a risk of failing to monitor patients' clinical conditions satisfactorily if we ignore the scanning and sorting capacity of computers but there are even greater risks when we lose sight of human beings in a blur of numbers.

Poor communication with colleagues

Communication skills are a vital part of all clinical practice. What we actually communicate is what arrives in the patient's mind rather than what we thought we said or did. When patients are frightened or unwell, they may not hear or remember things as well as they would normally do. Doctors therefore need to repeat ourselves, write things down, use other staff to reinforce what we said, and use any number of techniques to help patients to understand their clinical conditions and what we have suggested for them. It is no good saying "But I told him ...". We may have done so – but the information did not arrive and therefore the communication did not occur.

Doctors are responsible for the work of our secretaries and other staff. It is all very well in politically correct circles for the assumption to be made that the doctor is not necessarily the head of the clinical team. That is frankly bizarre. Someone has to be responsible for overall clinical management and for accurate communication. If people want to take over this responsibility from doctors then perhaps they should train to become doctors. For doctors themselves to delegate responsibility for their communications is completely unacceptable.

Communication between hospital and general medical practice tends to be a disaster area. Even in these days of computers, photocopiers, faxes and telephones, it can still take weeks to get information from hospitals. Yet specialists in these same hospitals often expect a letter in the hand or even in advance of the patient arriving in their clinics. This problem can be solved by shared computerised records but there is inevitably some loss of confidentiality in that process. Patients need to be aware of that, but we must hope that they will come to understand that there is an inevitable trade-off between better clinical care and the loss of some level of confidentiality. Again, Professor Lawrence Weed is at the forefront of clinical understanding on these issues. His book, *Medical Education, Medical Records and Patient Care* (Yearbook Publications 1969) is still the seminal work on the subject, more than thirty years after it was first published.

Ethical Failures

The final group of mistakes that can cause physical harm to patients comes as a result of doctors' ethical failures.

Falsifying records

As I have emphasised repeatedly, we all make mistakes. On discovering them we should do what we can to correct them but certainly not falsify the records. There is no shame whatever in acknowledging a mistake but there should be a great deal of shame attached to trying to pretend that we never made the mistake in the first place.

It always amazes me when professors get caught falsifying the data in their research studies. Becoming a professor requires many years of hard work built upon natural skills. Why on earth would all this be jeopardised for the sake of a particular research paper? I assume that kudos and money are major influences in this corrupt process - but how sordid and pathetic that is. At a less exalted level of clinical practice, general medical practitioners and hospital doctors are sometimes caught falsifying research projects on behalf of drug companies, or they may falsify other administrative or clinical documents for financial gain. Again, one would hope that doctors, of all people, would see the dangers to their patients of falsifying data and see the risks to themselves of getting involved in fraudulent activities. But often they don't - and they finish up in front of the General Medical Council disciplinary committee with monotonous regularity.

Abusing professional relationships

The tabloid press makes great play on the sexual relationships between doctors and their patients. The extreme cases get into the newspapers because that is what some newspapers like to print. However, this is not a universal practice even though it is much more common than might be imagined. I once heard the estimate that one in five of all doctors have had sexual contact of one kind or another with a patient. I suppose one should not be surprised because the most frequent human contact that doctors ever experience is with their patients. Even so, that is no excuse: doctors betray the trust put in them when they have sexual contact of any kind with their patients. (Incidentally, this applies as much to female doctors as to their male colleagues.)

Financial dealings with patients are equally fraught with danger. I remember, from my early days in general practice, when I was covering another doctor's practice, I found a notice on his desk announcing to all his patients, in the relatively impoverished area in which he worked in comparison to the one in which he lived, "Your doctor is a bit short at the moment. Please would you lend him a few pounds?". It seems absolutely extraordinary - but it really did happen. There is nothing wrong in financial arrangements between two people if both are equally financially astute and if there is no likelihood of inappropriate pressures upon their relationship if things do not work out as expected financially. However, when the two people involved are doctor and patient, it must be a rare occasion when the professional relationship can be safeguarded.

Perhaps the most serious but least recorded abuse – at any rate in the popular press – is poor clinical standards. Twenty-five years ago I was asked to write an article for a national newspaper on the subject of the need for GPs to have postgraduate education. Within the article I wrote about the need for them to have washbasins in their offices. At the time a survey had shown that 20% of NHS GPs consulting rooms had no washbasins and therefore appropriate clinical examination of their patients was well nigh impossible. The article was rejected. It is extraordinary how generally tolerant the press and even patients themselves can be of sloppy standards. The touching faith expressed by patients in their doctor's capacity to be "an excellent diagnostician" seems often to be totally without foundation. Normal judgement has been suspended.

Occasionally doctors will cause deliberate harm to their patients. These are criminal acts and should be treated as such. In this respect the boundary between ethical clinical research and deliberate harm can at times be disturbingly vague.

The sick doctor

Doctors have the same physical illnesses as other people and they also have the same mental illnesses as the general population. It has been estimated that one in ten of the population in general, including doctors, have problems with alcohol or drugs. It is known that five doctors are usually involved in one way or another when a patient has a surgical operation. Putting these two figures together it would appear that the chances of one of the doctors involved in a surgical operation being addicted to alcohol or drugs are 50%. Obviously one has to interpret these figures cautiously and one cannot extrapolate from the general to the particular. Nonetheless, we should be far more aware of this problem than we tend to be.

Doctors also have the same prejudices as the general population. It always amazes me when this comes to light because doctors, of all people, are in at the beginning and end of their patients' lives and therefore have practical experience of the equality of mankind in these fundamental processes. Nonetheless, the fact is that we can be just as bigoted as anyone else and this has obvious dangers for our patients.

Doctors becoming Gods

As a general rule, when doctors ask patients to do something, they do it. We ask patients to stick out their tongues or touch their toes or take their clothes off and they do. This power can be very seductive. Sometimes we expect people to bow low before us – or certainly to listen to our opinions – simply *because* we are doctors. Sometimes we do things to a patient more because we *can* do them rather than because we have really thought about whether they are absolutely in the patient's best interest. We get carried away with our power and we lose sight of the trust that has been placed in us and the privilege and responsibility we have in caring for others. This is unacceptable.

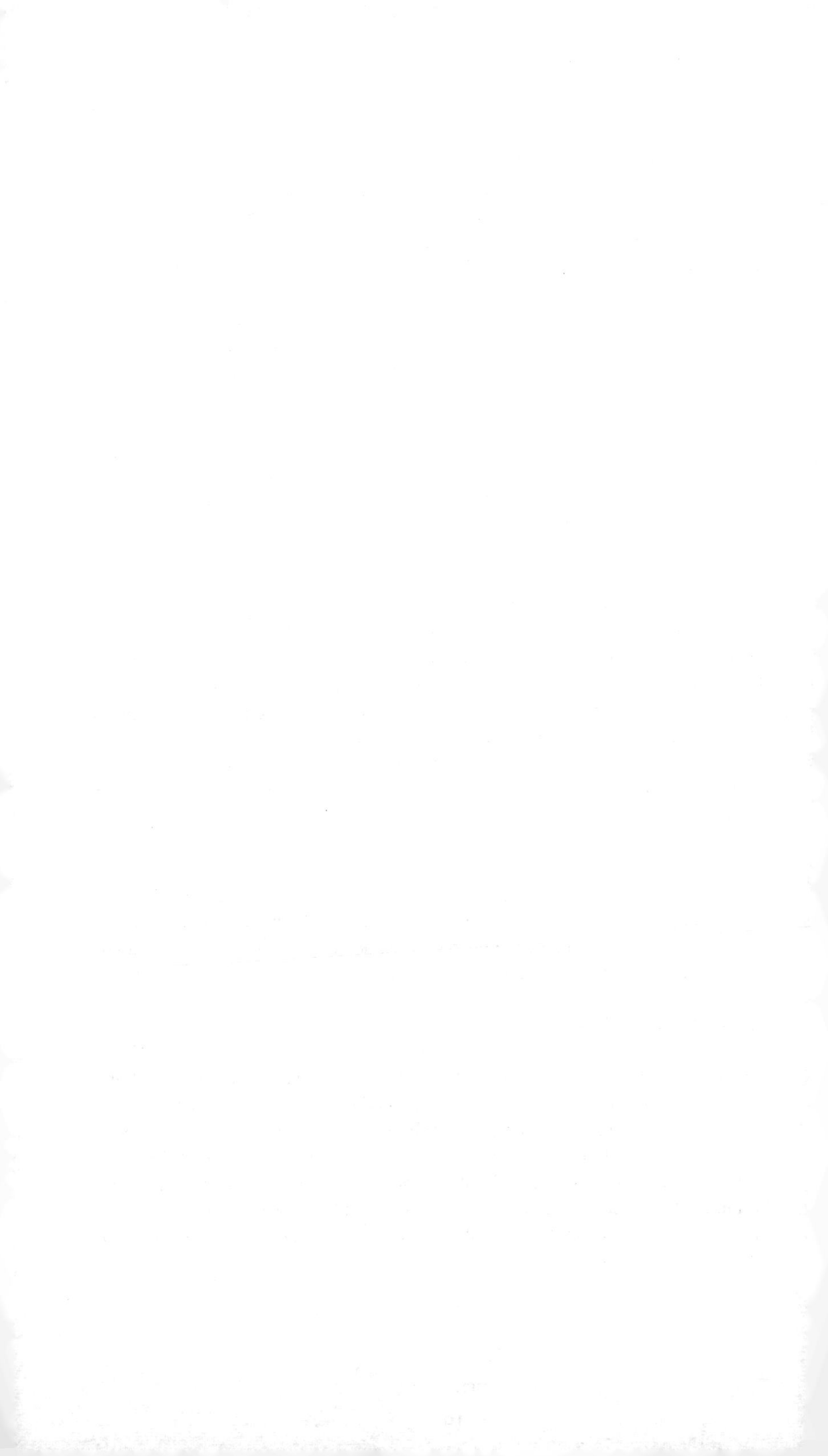

Chapter Three

Patients' Contributions to Doctors' Mistakes

Patients can never be blamed for the actions of their doctors. Nonetheless, there are circumstances in which the patient's own actions can be a contributory factor when examining the damaging behaviour of doctors.

Sometimes patients have Utopian expectations with no understanding of time pressures or the limit in resources of staff, equipment and financial capacity available to their doctors. Politicians and the press may have raised their hopes, but they themselves may have expectations that are simply impossible to fulfil. Patients may read or hear about particular medical advances and not realise that these are not immediately available or that they are not necessarily appropriate. The pressure group culture that has infected our society has resulted in people demanding progressively more for themselves while expecting that other, often unspecified, people should provide for them. The assumption may be that "rich" people should pay more – regardless of the evidence that they simply stop producing when they find that it is not worth their while to do so – and patients and their pressure groups may expect the Government to channel resources towards their particular concerns. These patients and pressure groups may like to believe that the Utopian situation of universal welfare has already arrived. It has not – but that will not make any difference to the demands on politicians, or the offers made by some of them at election times.

The sad thing is that patients who genuinely need the most help are often those who are least complaining. They may be extraordinarily grateful for what they are given, whereas other people, with far lesser need, complain incessantly that they are not given enough.

There is also a rather strange belief that doctors will do good work to order. I remember some patients complaining when I resigned from the NHS that they would no longer be able to hold over my head the threat of reporting me to the authorities. I was taken aback that they could be quite so honest in acknowledging their motivation. It had never occurred to me that some of the people that I had looked after for years valued the power of government to coerce me. In my innocence, I thought that I was giving something of my own free will and that this might even have been appreciated. I am sure it was by the vast majority of my patients – but the others left a nasty taste in my mouth when considering the nature of state-funded systems of medical care.

On the other hand, private systems of medical care tend to be haunted by fears of litigation. Lawyers rule and nothing untoward can happen without them seeing an opportunity for litigation and compensation. In both systems – state or private – doctors can be hunted. They cannot possibly do their best work under such circumstances and it must be more likely that they will make mistakes. Furthermore, defensive medical practice is expensive – because doctors do too much for fear of being accused of doing too little – and it can be slow and dangerous. Obviously there have to be checks and balances on doctors' actions but there are sensible limits beyond which they become counter-productive.

Sometimes patients can be inconsiderate to their doctors both personally and professionally. This is obviously unacceptable but it has to be remembered by doctors that patients may behave that way particularly when they are ill or frightened. The remarkable thing is that patients are as considerate as they are in these circumstances. Even so, there are occasions when some patients would try the patience of Job.

Patients as their own Worst Advocates

Pests

For patients to be concerned about their symptoms is totally understandable. For them to be worried and confused so that they don't hear properly what is said to them is also understandable. For them to go on and on asking the same question and making the same demand is another matter altogether. Browbeating may be acceptable (although I question that) for television interviewers or parliamentary debaters but this process is now becoming part of our general culture and we are all the worse for it.

Diagnostic fixation

Sometimes patients get an absolutely rigid belief that their symptoms are due to a particular cause – and nothing will shift them from that belief. The sad thing is that sometimes they are right; but their method of going about trying to persuade doctors of the truth of their perceptions can at times be almost guaranteed to achieve the opposite of considerate care. As doctors, we must learn that the perpetual complaint does have to be clinically investigated properly but, at the same time, it may be an indication of a psychological problem. This of course is exactly what the patient does not want us to consider – but it may nonetheless be true.

I remember a man believing that I had killed his daughter by prescribing a contraceptive pill for her and causing a pulmonary thrombosis. He telephoned me at 2.00 am night after night to call me a murderer. I had not in fact prescribed the contraceptive pill for her at all and the post mortem examination showed that she died of Hodgkin's disease. I never heard from the man again and would not expect to do so. He probably still believes that I gave her the contraceptive pill and that it, in some way, gave rise to or aggravated her Hodgkin's disease. The pain of his loss would cause him to search for reasons – any reasons whatever. I was simply in his firing line and there was nothing I could do to get out of it.

That experience happens to all doctors at some time and we simply have to accept that it goes with the job in the same way that occasionally people will treat us as gods. We cannot accept one extreme while rejecting the other.

More commonly patients who are chronically tired may believe that they have a particular medical condition, such as M.E., and believe that there is a medical conspiracy to prevent this diagnosis – or whatever they have in mind – being more widely accepted. Again, all that doctors can do in these circumstances is simply to carry out the appropriate clinical examination and investigations and state our findings and our beliefs. If patients don't agree with us, then at least we know that we have done our best. It is clinically appropriate to look at other possible causes of the patient's tiredness – particularly emotional causes – but, again, patients may resist that, sometimes vehemently.

The "worried well", who are absolutely convinced that they have vitamin or trace element deficiencies, food allergies, intestinal candidiasis and a host of other weird and wonderful diagnoses that have little or no scientific merit, and when there is no clinical evidence of the condition, can be the bread and butter of some private doctors. Personally, I find these patients and their doctors painful in the extreme. Healthy living and a healthy diet should be a universal, rather than medical, responsibility except in extreme circumstances. Similarly, I find that "fibromyalgia", pelvic tilts as a result of one leg being shorter than the other, osteoarthrosis (whatever that might be), mal-aligned discs, fibrous "knots" and various other pseudo-diagnoses sometimes used by osteopaths, chiropractors and other "specialists in orthopaedic medicine" leave me cold. Very often I like what these professionals do to their patients – because I believe that simple mechanical treatments are much preferable to long-term medications or unnecessary surgical operations – but I do wish that they would get on with their practical procedures and keep their mouths shut.

In this respect patients are often their own worst enemies when they demand a diagnosis. Yet again, Professor Lawrence Weed shows the way by insisting that "pain" is a perfectly reasonable diagnosis in its own right. Trying to specify its cause when we have no adequate scientific evidence simply complicates the issue and may lead us down the wrong diagnostic and therapeutic path altogether.

The emotional component of any illness

However reluctant patients may be to accept that there is an emotional component to their symptoms, the fact is that this is true in all circumstances. All that is up for discussion is the significance of that particular component in any particular circumstance. The word "psychosomatic" has not been helpful in this respect. *All* clinical conditions affect both the body and the mind, just as they affect one's social function to some extent. Diagnoses should therefore be considered not simply in physical terms but also in psychological, mental and social terms. It has taken doctors many centuries to re-learn this approach that was known to the ancient Greeks and probably to many other ancient cultures before them. It should be no surprise that patients also find it difficult to accept the concept of broadly based, rather than single specific, diagnosis.

At times doctors may be very inconsiderate towards patients' emotional problems. We tend not to be trained at all in medical school for this aspect of our work and some doctors find themselves personally very ill-equipped to deal with it. When we consider that all consultations in general medical practice have some emotional component and that it is the primary component in one third of the consultations, we realise the total inadequacy of medical education in this respect. By seeing these patients as "nuisances" or as being "pathetic", doctors may be totally underestimating the severity of their patients' problems. Emotional issues can be just as debilitating as physical issues and they are just as worthy of our understanding and care.

Patients who are mentally ill can also have a very bad time at the hands of doctors on some occasions. People suffering from paranoid schizophrenia, who believe they have enemies, are more than capable of making enemies as a result – and sadly, some of these enemies are their own doctors. That is unacceptable, and again reflects inadequate focus on this issue during undergraduate medical education.

"Professional" knowledge of the patient

Patients may sometimes think that they know more than the doctor. Sometimes they may be right. They may have looked up a subject on the Internet or read an article in the press and therefore be bang up-to-date on the subject of interest to them. For doctors to be equally up-to-date in absolutely every subject is totally impossible. At times we therefore have to learn to be humble, read what the patient sends us and make a judgement on its relevance.

This humbling process is fine in theory but does not always work out well in practice. I receive several articles from patients every week – in addition to a vast quantity of medical literature sent to me in free medical periodicals and from the Department of Health. I do read the articles sent to me by patients but the catch comes when I disagree with the patient's view of them.

Recently I found a man in his 50s had a raised blood test result for the level of prostate-specific antigen. This can happen with simple inflammation but can also be an early sign of cancer. Some differentiation between these two possibilities comes from looking at the ratio between the "free" and "total" fractions of the prostate-specific antigen. The issue of precise interpretation of the blood test result is complex: there is no simple yes/no answer. Further tests such as a prostatic biopsy (taking a sample of the prostate gland through a tube inserted into the rectum) may be necessary. The age of the patient is relevant because it is reckoned that surgical treatment would not necessarily give a greater expectation of life in some elderly patients – and for that reason it would be contra-indicated. The risks of surgery leading to impotence or incontinence or other complications are significant and should not be taken lightly. Financial considerations over the cost of the test or of surgery may also play a part.

In the UK, the current policy of the Department of Health is that the prostate-specific antigen test should not be performed as a routine screening procedure but should only be taken when the patient has specific symptoms that might raise the diagnostic possibility of cancer of the prostate. In the USA, with its greater incidence of litigation, that policy would be unacceptable. On that same basis, colonoscopic examination for malignancies in the colon are commonplace screening procedures in the USA but are generally not done as part of a routine health check in the UK.

The specialist to whom I referred particular the patient with the raised prostate-specific antigen found no further abnormality on further investigation. The patient then consulted an NHS doctor who said that I should never have done the test in the first place nor referred him for specialist opinion. In my view the first point is debatable (although I stick to my policy of doing a routine screening test for prostate-specific antigen in men above the age of 45) but the second point is not. I cannot sit on an abnormal test result and not refer it for further opinion to a specialist urologist. Correspondence between the patient and me, together with photocopies of supporting articles, went backwards and forwards for three weeks with neither of us shifting our opinion.

My own view is that it is fair enough for patients to challenge my clinical opinion. Nonetheless, it does sometimes surprise me when they reject my professional opinion for the personal viewpoint of someone sitting next to them at a dinner party. In this respect the choice of consultant specialist is something that the patient will very often announce to me on the basis "my friend tells me that I must see so and so ...". I have learnt from experience that there is no point in fighting a battle of that nature: I simply give up the unequal struggle and make the referral to the specialist requested by the patient rather than to the one whom I know and have learned to trust.

Personal experience with the illness of a friend or family member can sometimes give patients a very fixed viewpoint on what should be done for their own condition. It is difficult to argue against "My aunt had that operation and it killed her" or "All my friends swear by vitamin B12 injections". To some extent doctors have to be philosophical about this problem: patients have a right to their own idiosyncrasies and beliefs. On the other hand it would be unethical as well as dangerous to accept that patients should automatically have the right to determine the course of action that doctors should take. Although I work in the private sector and risk upsetting my patients when I refuse to do their bidding, I do not prescribe tranquillisers or anti-depressants, let alone vitamin B12 injections (except where they are specifically necessary in the treatment of pernicious anaemia).

In private practice, the process of sticking to one's own beliefs as a doctor means that you eventually end up with a whole list of patients who agree with those beliefs – because the others leave and go elsewhere. I believe that process to be perfectly appropriate. For this reason, among others, I would never consider having a committee of patients to advise me on either the structure of the services that I should supply (such as baby clinics or chiropody services) or on the treatments that I should prescribe. My own practical principle, "If you don't like me, find someone else to look after you", may seem arrogant and dictatorial but I believe it to be common sense. When drug addicts demand a prescription of Methadone from me,

I simply refuse. I do not believe in that form of "treatment" for heroin addiction. I give those patients the name of a doctor who does. To be answerable to my patients in general clinical and ethical terms does not mean that they have the right to dictate what I should do. I believe that it is perfectly acceptable for Roman Catholic doctors to refuse to refer patients for termination of pregnancy and that it is perfectly reasonable for them to discuss alternatives with the patients. Even so the patient does not have the right to insist that the doctor makes the referral and the doctor does not have the right to insist that the patient should *not* seek a further opinion from someone else.

These issues seem relatively straightforward to me but I know from experience that they can become remarkably complicated when the Department of Health decides that a particular issue should be government policy. In a recent case a private general practitioner was hauled before the General Medical Council because he advised his patients to have separate inoculations for measles, mumps and rubella rather than the combined MMR vaccine because he believed that there might be some truth in the report that the combined vaccine could lead to a possible increase in autism. The Government case was that there are very significant risks of measles epidemics – leading to mortality as well as morbidity – if the overall pool of vaccinated children falls below the epidemiologically critical level of 85%. The doctor's case was that he was answering a perceived need of his patients. Both sides have a point. In the event, the case against the doctor collapsed and the worst fears of the Department of Health were realised when the uptake of MMR did indeed fall below 85% and the risk of outbreaks of measles reappeared. At present it is still impossible to decide, on the available evidence, whether the doctor in question was irresponsible in putting children at risk of measles or responsible in protecting them from autism. I suspect the former, even though the correctness of Government epidemiological policies on BSE, foot and mouth disease and even AIDS has been highly questionable.

Ultimately I believe that the press has a great deal to answer for on medical issues such as these. They love medical scare stories. I suppose we get the press that we deserve, just as we get the doctors that we deserve.

In the Western world there are few places where patients have no choice other than to see a particular doctor or where doctors have no choice but to see a particular patient. NHS doctors are allowed to have patients removed from their lists but also sometimes have to accept other patients being allocated to them. I myself never removed any patients from my NHS list except when the local health authority insisted on one occasion that I had too many patients. However, over the years, I quite often had patients allocated to me when other doctors had them removed from their lists. Most commonly I found that the reason that doctors had removed these patients was not because they were chronically sick or old and infirm or that they were mentally ill, but because they were "know-it-alls".

Deliberate Harm to the Doctor

Violence with or without weapons

It would appear from newspapers and, in particular, from medical magazines that violence against doctors, especially against general medical practitioners, is becoming increasingly common in the UK. A published photograph of various weapons that have been used against doctors in the last year was certainly very alarming. One has to remember that GPs are in the front line in society's battle against drugs and in society's concern for people who are mentally ill.

Hospital Accident and Emergency Departments are even more exposed. It is estimated that 50% of patients attending Accident and Emergency Departments are there as a result of some form of problem caused by the use of alcohol or drugs. Doctors, nurses, ambulance men and women and even administrative staff can sometimes pay a heavy price for their professional commitment. On the mental wards, episodes of violence against staff are a major concern because of their sheer frequency as well as ferocity.

The general public are informed with commendable clarity and frequency when the behaviour of doctors and other healthcare professionals towards their patients falls below acceptable standards. Violence against healthcare professionals rarely makes the news except when doctors or other medical staff are murdered in the course of their work. The same is true for teachers, probation officers, social workers, the police and anyone else involved in the various front lines of society's battles. It is almost as if the risk of violence is now taken for granted as part of the job. This is an appalling state of affairs but it is difficult to know what can be done about it. However, if New York City can pull itself together under a policy of zero tolerance imposed by a non-liberal mayor, then so could the rest of the world. We have perhaps become too tolerant and understanding. It is strange indeed when the perpetrators of crimes are portrayed as victims.

I live and work in a privileged area of London and my former home in North Kensington was burgled three times. My general medical practice premises, however, have never been burgled or vandalised. I do not stock controlled drugs other than in minimal quantities because I very rarely prescribe them so there is nothing worth taking in that respect. It is known "on the street" that I don't prescribe addictive drugs and it is also known that I will do everything I possibly can to help people to come off them. I believe that it is this reputation that keeps my premises relatively trouble-free. The one drunken patient who threw a glass ornament at my secretary was promptly arrested when I called the police. I too believe in zero tolerance of this sort of behaviour.

Last year I was asked by a researcher from the Royal College of Psychiatrists if our addiction treatment centre would like to send staff to a seminar on violence in psychiatric institutions. I explained that in seventeen years of operation, in which we have treated over three thousand inpatients, many of whom live in London and have come from very under-privileged backgrounds, we have had no significant episodes of violence against staff. Again I believe that this is precisely because we stock and prescribe very few drugs. The psychological profiles of our inpatients show them to be more disturbed than the average in-patient in psychiatric hospitals. Yet still we have no significant episodes of violence. By and large, I believe that when patients are treated with respect and dignity, on an in-patient basis or anywhere else, they respond in like manner. When people are drugged out of their minds with pharmaceutical or illegal substances then there is no knowing how they will behave.

Analysis of doctors' prescribing habits show that in the UK over forty million prescriptions for anti-depressants, tranquillisers or sleeping tablets are written each year. This is an appalling indictment of doctors' clinical attitudes and I believe it comes directly as a result of the obsession in medical schools that they should train doctors in the use of pharmaceutical substances. We are trained to prescribe rather than to listen, let alone care.

The policy of the Department of Health on treating heroin addicts with regular prescriptions of the oral substitute Methadone is equally misguided. The idea behind this policy is that addicts who are given a regular supply of a pharmaceutical liquid will not be tempted into crime to obtain their mood-altering drug and will not risk spreading AIDS and hepatitis B and C into the general population via sexual activity or the use of contaminated needles. This policy is patently absurd. In the first case, a study by *The Big Issue*, which is a responsible social organisation particularly concerned with the homeless, showed that 50% of all people taking regular Methadone were augmenting this with daily heroin obtained illegally. The policy of Methadone maintenance is fatally flawed because it simply does not work in keeping people away from illegal substances. It is comparable to giving alcoholics a few pints of free beer in the hope of keeping them out of the bar.

More cynically I believe that the policy of Methadone maintenance is financially and socially motivated: Methadone maintenance is cheap whereas treatment programmes are expensive. Furthermore, providing treatment for addicts so that they are guided towards total abstinence has to start from the belief that these patients are capable of achieving that outcome and that they are worth the effort. I know from seventeen years of clinical experience of running a Minnesota Method treatment centre that these patients very much deserve the right to be treated for addictive disease in the same way as they would deserve to be treated for diabetes, heart disease or cancer. Our outcome studies show that 65% of our patients are either totally abstinent or significantly improved (having had one or two short relapses) one year after leaving treatment. Despite this evidence, and similar evidence from other Minnesota Method treatment centres throughout the world, the Department of Health remains stubbornly resistant to providing Minnesota Method treatment within the NHS. Perhaps this resistance is based upon clinical doubt as to whether the outcome really is as successful as repeated studies have shown. Perhaps it is financial, recognising that the short-term costs of treatment are high and the outcome not guaranteed. Perhaps it is social, believing that addicts are not worth treating in the first place. Perhaps it is habitual, believing that the first line of attack against any clinical condition should always be pharmaceutical.

Whatever the reason, there are no Minnesota Method treatment centres of any stature within the entire NHS in the UK. The concept of "addictive disease" is generally dismissed and addiction is still seen as being a product of weak will, depravity and foolish experiment. There are none so blind as politicians, policy-makers, civil servants and doctors who simply *will* not see. I suspect that one reason for this is the sheer hassle and grief caused by alcoholics, drug addicts and other sufferers from addictive disease in one form or another. They give doctors and other healthcare workers a very hard time indeed, just as they do to everyone else. It is small wonder that the policy of pacifying them with Methadone, tranquillisers, anti-depressants and almost anything, should be so popular.

Occasionally patients who have no mental or addictive problem whatever will, nonetheless, inflict deliberate harm upon their doctors when they feel frustrated as a result of not being given treatment that they believe they deserve. This is essentially a political issue. It comes as a direct result of the belief that people have more rights than responsibilities. If a political or philosophical idea is rotten to the core, then it is small wonder that the behaviour that emanates from it will also be rotten.

Theft and burglary

Petty crime – and sometimes not so petty – is nowadays targeted as much against doctors as against anyone else. Just as there is a widespread belief that robbing a bank or defrauding the Inland Revenue are not "real" crimes because they are against institutions rather than individuals, correspondingly NHS premises, equipment and supplies appear to be thought of as "fair game" because they belong to the Government.

Thefts and burglaries are not always in pursuit of drugs or medications or of equipment that could be sold in exchange for drugs. Sometimes the thefts are simply opportunistic, and burglaries and vandalism may simply be part of an entitlement culture or part of the belief system of an "under-class".

These problems are much more deep-rooted than anything to do with doctors and the services that they provide. The problems – and their potential solutions – are political.

Emotional pressure

There is emotional pressure in any job, particularly in those where there is a direct interface with the general public. Now that parliamentary debate and television "chat shows" have degenerated into slanging matches, a new norm has been established: the public pressure group and the individual harangue are nowadays the "gold standard" of communication. If you want something done, you have to shout and complain and pile on the pressure. The vast majority of patients do not behave in this way but the few who do can be exceedingly troublesome.

Harassment by the Government is much more troublesome and exceedingly difficult to counter. As a result, the British Medical Association has become far more of a trade union than a professional organisation. It fights the doctors' corner against the Government. It often does so in the name of "improving services to patients" but, more realistically, the B.M.A. directives can usually be seen in the same light as those of any trade union, demanding "more pay for less work". In this poisoned atmosphere, exacerbated every week in the medical periodicals, particularly those sent free to doctors, it is small wonder that doctors become bitter and resentful and hence even lazy and incompetent. Those who resign from the NHS and go into full-time private practice sometimes discover that this option is not as easy as they might have anticipated. Private patients expect the three "As": availability, affability and ability, in that order of significance. More commonly, doctors retain their NHS appointments – and the various privileges and expenses that go with them – and do some private work "on the side". Sometimes this is done honourably with private practice making inroads into personal rather than professional time but commonly it is the other way round and NHS patients get a raw deal both in hospital and in general practice when doctors work both for the State and in pursuit of their own private practice.

One way or the other, and for one reason or another, there is nowadays considerable emotional pressure upon doctors. Even those of us who work exclusively privately are ultimately answerable, as we should be, to the State. Those of us who run private institutions find the red tape of health authority supervision absolutely exasperating. The greatest fear of civil servants is that they themselves will be held responsible for anything that goes wrong in a private institution under their supervision. As a result, regulations that were originally designed simply as guidelines become cast in stone with results that are sometimes simply ludicrous. For example, in our addiction treatment centre our patients are generally young and physically fit, yet the bedrooms all have to have ceiling heights capable of accommodating bed hoists. The reason for this is that our treatment centre comes under the same set of regulations as those for old people's homes – and so far there has been absolutely no room for latitude or sensible interpretation of those regulations.

All bureaucracy works with the same blind determination, with the civil servants dreading being caught holding the parcel when the music stops. The problem is far from unique in medical services. Nonetheless, the end result is often that patients do not get the services that they could receive because it is simply not worth the money or the hassle for the proprietors to provide them. Proprietors of private medical institutions are often portrayed as being avaricious and even seedy and there is a general belief in the broadly socialist culture of the welfare state in the UK that people should not "make profits from the sick". The end result is that the provision of private nursing homes has decreased dramatically in recent years and this has had a knock-on effect on acute hospitals where the beds become blocked by patients who have nowhere to go if they are too frail to be returned to their own homes. Of course there have to be regulations and of course there are abuses that have to be corrected – but very often the first casualty of bureaucracy is common sense.

Occasionally the patients themselves put deliberate emotional pressure upon doctors in the hope that they will get better service as a result. Surely the opposite must be the case: the doctor may indeed provide the service on this occasion – but he or she will never forget being pressurised and that is bound to affect his or her clinical practice and personal attitudes at some time in the future.

Patients become frustrated when they believe that they are not getting the services to which they are entitled. On occasions this frustration is perfectly justified. There are indeed lazy and incompetent doctors and the medical profession could indeed do more to weed them out. However, there are difficulties with universal legislation when the regulations are formulated so tightly that they can catch anyone at some time or other. All doctors make mistakes. "Naming and shaming" us – as happened in 2001 to one doctor who was mentioned by name in a parliamentary debate – is not constructive. The adversarial attitude of some health managers – one Health Authority Chairman has been known openly to describe doctors as "the enemy" – is not exactly helpful. The odds are even: some doctors are dreadful and so are some Health Authority officials – but others on both sides are very good. The problem comes when regulations and policies designed to weed out or improve the bad have the unintentional – but perhaps inevitable – result of hindering the good. Under these circumstances, any doctor can become resentful when pressurised by patients' demands for better services, particularly when the doctors themselves may have minimal influence upon the provision of those services.

Self-harm

Patients are understandably worried about their medical ailments. They can be totally vulnerable and absolutely powerless in the hands of doctors and other healthcare professionals if they are to get appropriate diagnosis and treatment and hence be able to return to normal function. Some patients are their own worst enemies in this respect by becoming so worried about one little thing after another that doctors become exasperated. In general medical practice one learns – or should do – that these patients have a "dis-ease" that is no less significant than many named diseases. These patients are certainly debilitated. They tend to get diagnosed as having "neurotic ill health" and prescribed tranquillisers, anti-depressants or other mood-altering drugs. This is a clinical disaster of the first order. The patients can be helped in many ways other than pharmaceutically and they deserve better understanding and treatment than that.

At the extreme, Munchausen's syndrome, in which patients produce one medical condition after another and even fabricate them so that they get almost constant medical attention and finish up having multiple treatments, including surgical operations, is totally debilitating. These patients are sometimes seen as "trouble" for the medical profession. Alcoholics and drug addicts and people who suffer from other forms of compulsive behaviour are also often seen in that light. The truth is that these patients have illnesses that are just as worthy of understanding by the medical profession and just as capable of appropriate treatment once the conditions and those who suffer from them are seen in the proper light. Far from wasting doctors' time or being a nuisance or squandering scarce resources, these patients need to be accurately diagnosed and sensitively treated. Their problems are primarily psychological rather than physical – although there may be physical consequences – but these patients deserve to be treated with the same respect and dignity as any other.

Self-mutilation by patients can be exasperating for general medical practitioners or doctors and nurses working in Accident and Emergency Departments but again this "dis-ease" needs to be seen – and treated – in psychological terms. Self-mutilation is often seen in patients who suffer from dissociative identity disorder (in which two or more different parts of the patient's personality inhabit the same body but behave very differently) and this is commonly seen in people who have had horrendously abusive childhoods. Far from being criticised or even scorned and dismissed, these patients – more than most – deserve our sympathy and skill: sewing up their wounds is only the first, and least significant thing we can do for them.

"Depression" often leads to patients becoming severely incapacitated. Their whole lives fall apart. For doctors to respond by prescribing one "anti-depressant" after another in the guise of "help" is tragic. These patients deserve far better treatment than "a pill for every ill". This medication may "work" – but only in the same way that heroin would work for toothache: something may be done for the symptom but nothing for the underlying condition. Furthermore, anti-depressants and other mood-altering drugs trap the patients in a very narrow band of capacity for creativity and human interchange. Enthusiasm and creativity die. It is small wonder that anti-depressants are commonly used in overdose by successful suicides. There are many ways of treating "depression" other than through the use of pharmaceutical medications. These alternative methods should surely be the first approach rather than the last. Our patients deserve better than medications.

Interestingly, a recent, carefully controlled study (Andrew F. Leuchter and others: *American Journal of Psychiatry 2002:159:122-129*) showed that patients are sometimes their own worst enemies when they demand medication. In this study, depressed patients were divided into two groups. One group was treated with the latest selective Serotonin re-uptake inhibitor (SSRI) anti-depressant and the other group was treated with a capsule that appeared identical but which contained a sugar rather than any form of drug. Neither the patients nor the doctor knew which patients were receiving the drug or the sugar. At the end of the study it was found that many patients who had been taking the sugar had done just as well as those who had been taking the drug. This was no great surprise because the "placebo effect", in which patients do well when they trust the doctor or the therapeutic process, is well known. What was surprising – and fascinating – is that all but one of the patients taking the sugar relapsed back to their former depressed state when they discovered that they had been taking a sugar. They then demanded to be given a real medicine. The one exceptional patient noted appropriately that if benefit occurred from taking a sugar then there was no indication for taking a drug. What this study indicates to me is that patients often want to take prescription drugs, just as doctors want to prescribe them, because the medications establish the "sick" state rather than one of personal responsibility for disturbed feelings.

Even when the patients are demanding "a pill for every emotional ill", their doctors should stand firm and help them to see that their own values and personal philosophy and behaviour are the most likely cause of their symptoms (once purely physical causes such as anaemia or thyroid deficiency have been ruled out). Generally patients respond well when they are given time and understanding and an opportunity to talk about their difficulties. It does not have to be the doctor's own ear that listens – there are many other professionals trained to listen – but it helps if it is. After all, what is it that doctors really want to do with their lives – examine sore throats and skin rashes? I do not belittle these clinical conditions but I do believe that emotional conditions are even more worthy of the doctor's time than physical conditions – because they are so far-reaching in their effects. When people are distraught they tend to smoke and drink too much and do all sorts of other things that are damaging to themselves and others. Ultimately these behaviours result in physical damage and also result in widespread knock-on effects in the family and at work and sometimes in society at large.

Surely it is better for doctors to be in at the beginning of this process rather than to wait until the damage has been done before stepping forward and saying "I am a doctor. Can I help?". Doctors may believe that it is the patient's fault when they get medical conditions that are the consequence of their own self-destructive behaviour. Perhaps, going further back in time than that, it is the doctor's fault for not listening when the patient cried for help on the first occasion. I myself believe that the provision of this listening service should be the *primary* responsibility of doctors in general medical practice, alongside equipping themselves with appropriate diagnostic facilities to enable them to make early diagnosis of significant physical disease. Infant inoculations, monitoring of high blood pressure and diabetes and attending to the elderly, the chronically sick and disabled are all functions that can be managed perfectly well, and responsibly carried out, by appropriately trained and experienced nursing staff.

If patients, through their own actions, sometimes make life difficult for doctors, that is just the way it is. It is part of their "dis-ease" and it is up to us doctors to find ways to help them.

Chapter Four

Mental Illness Created by Doctors

We are all of us aware of iatrogenic *physical* illness, those caused when doctors and other health workers damage patients in a physical way. Many untoward events and even hospital admissions may be due to doctors' errors or to the unintended results of their actions. We may be much less aware of widespread iatrogenic *mental* illness, dis-ease.

Emotional Dependency

"Thank you doctor, you are wonderful."

When patients say "Thank you, doctor, you are wonderful" the doctor should be concerned rather than flattered. "You have done a good piece of professional work" might be reasonable but "*you* are wonderful" is a different matter. The patient may be becoming emotionally dependent on the doctor, seeing him or her as a saviour rather than as a professional. Even more dangerous is when the doctor comes to believe it. Doctors who believe in their own brilliance and even invincibility can become very dangerous indeed when they don't see their own mistakes or, worse, bluster their way around them.

Patients may fail to see where they are being given sub-standard care. They lose their judgement and get taken in by appearance rather than convinced by substance. It is understandable that patients should want to believe in their doctors but it is dangerous for them to do so to such an extent that they lose all their reserve or judgement.

The unique power of doctors to prescribe medications tends to authenticate "the sick state" both in the patients' minds and in the minds of their doctors. With each prescription the doctor says "you are sick" and the patient, in taking it, believes it. Each takes his or her own position in the hierarchy of responsibility: the all-powerful doctor *versus* the supplicant patient. That relative position has considerable risks for both doctor and patient. Some doctors relish the power of prescription and prescribe more and more. They may believe that they are helping to such an extent that they fail to see both the physical risk and, sometimes even more importantly, the emotional risk of dependency. The doctor becomes a pharmaceutical tyrant, believing that all problems should be manageable with one medication or another. The patient becomes a pharmaceutical dependent, hoping that a pharmaceutical solution will always be available not only for physical problems but sometimes also for emotional, behavioural and social problems. It would be no bad thing if, for perhaps just one week in every year, all doctors were to put down their prescription pads altogether. They might see just how far they have come from caring for their patients in other ways – or even at all. Equally, their patients might come to see how much they themselves have become dependent upon the concept of "a pill for every ill". The doctor's power to prescribe and the patient's supplicant need for instant solutions to life's problems are both very seductive positions – and both equally destructive.

"My doctor is a wonderful diagnostician."

Patients will often say, "My doctor is a wonderful diagnostician". How on earth could they know? The point is that they *need* to believe that their doctor is a wonderful diagnostician because they know that if the diagnosis was wrong, then the treatment was wrong. It is not my purpose to undermine patients' confidence in their doctors but rather to encourage them to treat doctors' words with the same healthy scepticism that they would use for estate agents or politicians.

Occasionally patients will quote their doctors as saying something that they manifestly could not have said. For example, "My doctor said I had a cardiac heart" or "a gastric stomach". Cardiac means heart, gastric means stomach. No doctor would say that a patient had a heart heart or a stomach stomach. The point is that the patient *wants* a diagnosis that sounds important so that he or she feels that the suffering is due to a real condition and that he or she is not simply making a fuss. While this concern is understandable, it can also be very dangerous. Patients can become crippled by their own beliefs. Certainly "My doctor said that the inadequacies of my own personal philosophy are responsible for my behaviour and subsequently for a great many of my medical problems" does not have quite the same ring to it as "My doctor says I am not well at all". It may nonetheless be absolutely true and be exactly what the patient most *needs* to hear. However, I cannot imagine anyone ever *wanting* to hear that.

Thus, in the relationship between doctor and patient, there may be a predetermined agenda from both sides. The doctor may be saying "I have the knowledge and skill to be able to help you" and the patient may be saying "I need a doctor to authenticate my incapacity". It would be much healthier if each came with a totally different agenda with the doctor saying "I have very limited powers to help patients, and should say and do as little as is absolutely necessary and in the patient's best interests. I should not take responsibility *for* my patients but should be responsible *to* them". And the patient should say "I want to ask for my doctor's help solely for things that I cannot do for myself and will only take medication or treatment that enhances rather than reduces my capacity to be independent physically, emotionally and socially".

In fact emotional dependency is certainly not limited to patients' relationships with their doctors. The same can be true in any professional relationship: the electorate's relationship with politicians, pupils' relationship with teachers, the spiritually challenged in their relationship with the clergy. I believe that we delegate far too much to professionals. We should do our own thinking rather than delegate everything to politicians. Sometimes politicians take too much power simply because we give them too much power, because it is easy to blame them when things go wrong in our lives. We get the press we deserve because we choose to read smut and vitriol. We get the teachers we deserve because we don't value them sufficiently to pay them well. We get the clergy we deserve because we delegate all spiritual matters to them, believing (as they often do) that they have more direct lines of communication to God or to some other higher spiritual consciousness than we do.

We get the doctors we deserve when we fail to recognise how much we are responsible ourselves for our own health and well-being. In each case the abdication of personal responsibility brings disaster.

To say "my doctor is a wonderful diagnostician" is as incongruous as saying "this restaurant is the best Indian restaurant in London" when one has only been to a total of half a dozen. Saying "I like this particular doctor (or restaurant)" is fair enough. But the moment one closes one's mind to alternative possibilities, one is at the beginning of a very slippery slope. As far as preference for one restaurant over another is concerned, there is little disadvantage or risk. Closing one's mind to the prospect that there might be better doctors, however, would be daft – and potentially dangerous.

We tend to switch off our critical powers when we become *more* dependent upon the services that we are receiving. Thus, we may not be too bothered about whether we buy our food and clothing from one supermarket or mega-store or another. There will be some variations in price and quality but the decisions that we make are not absolutely vital. With motor mechanics the issue is not straightforward and will depend to some extent on how much we ourselves know about the workings of motor vehicles. It will also depend upon whether the vehicle itself is a standard run-about or a classic. When it comes to lawyers, architects, accountants, doctors and other professionals, we tend to act first of all on the recommendation of other people and secondly on whether we feel that there is a "fit" between our personalities and approach and theirs. Even then we may – quite rightly – challenge the opinion of a professional and want to see the evidence. However, by the time we are sitting in front of a Queen's Counsel or a brain surgeon we really don't have much choice but to listen to his or her opinion. It must be remembered that the most important decision made by a professional is the very first one on whether the client or patient has a problem in the first place. Thus, the professionals who first come in contact with the client – in the healthcare system, for example, GPs with patients – have a very considerable responsibility. For example, there is no chance of the patient having his brain tumour seen by a neurosurgeon at the right time if the GP's standard approach towards headaches is to say, without examining the patient, "This is migraine". The tragedy is that the *less* competent and thorough the professional approach of the doctor, the *more* likely it is that the patient will say "My doctor is a wonderful diagnostician" – because he or she really has no other choice but to believe that. When no evidence is given, the patient *has* to believe in the doctor's supernatural powers.

Judging the competence of a doctor – or lawyer or architect or teacher or politician or clergyman or anyone else – is not in fact as difficult as it sounds. Each of us will be just as good or bad in every aspect of our lives. If we are sloppy or unreliable or inefficient or if we jump to hasty conclusions, this will be apparent in *all* our relationships and in *all* aspects of our lives. On this basis, it is easy for us to observe the behaviour of a professional towards his or her staff or colleagues or family or other people in general, and deduce that we will be treated in exactly the same way.

If a doctor has a bleak waiting room, a grumpy receptionist and a messy desk, and if he or she looks scruffy and is unreliable with appointments and correspondence, then probably he or she is just as uncaring and unreliable in clinical matters. In such a case, to say "My doctor is a wonderful diagnostician" may be no more than wishful thinking.

Incorrect or Inadequate Diagnoses.

"Schizophrenia" or "paranoia"

These diagnoses may be used far too frequently, especially when thought disorders are drug-induced. Amphetamines, cocaine and other mood-altering drugs, including alcohol, can very commonly cause thought disorders. The correct approach is therefore to take patients off all substances first of all before making any diagnosis or considering prescribing anything at all.

When people have disturbances in their thought processes they can become exceedingly disruptive socially. I write as someone who has had his home burnt to the ground by a total stranger who now resides in a hospital for the criminally insane. Nonetheless, I am not convinced that schizophrenia or psychotic depression necessarily exist as clinical entities. Nor am I convinced that these patients should be treated with neuroleptic (anti-psychotic) medications. The newer generation of neuroleptic drugs are said to be more effective – or less dangerous – than their predecessors. However, it is instructive to realise just how far doctors are prepared to go. Neuroleptic drugs may control behaviour by damaging the brain, as can be seen in the frequent (40% or more in long-term use) incidence of tardive dyskinaesia (late development of increasing involuntary muscular movements) seen in patients taking the drugs most commonly prescribed in the last twenty years. Often these drug effects are wrongly thought to be part of the illness. Tardive akathisia (anxiety or nervousness and an uncontrollable desire to move the body) was seen in over 30% of the children who were prescribed these drugs. Nowadays these children would frequently be misdiagnosed as having attention deficit hyperactivity disorder – a condition of debatable existence. Tardive dementia (a progressive deterioration of the mind and mental faculties) can also occur, sometimes dramatically in "malignant" form. Neuroleptic drugs are prescribed to quieten patients and make them more manageable. From my personal and clinical experiences I might be thought to understand the temptation to prescribe out of vengeance but I do not. Treatment that damages the brain is wrong and there is no guarantee that the new generation of neuroleptic drugs will be found to be safer.

Dressing up the process of treatment in scientific language – noting the effect of the neurotransmitter dopamine in the emotion-regulating limbic system and frontal lobes of the brain – should not disguise what is being done to the human being. Cognitive behavioural approaches, motivational enhancement techniques and attempts to provide basic emotional and social support – even in prison, let alone in hospital or in the community – should be used in preference to drugs that might cause terrible destruction.

Nonetheless, even if a mental condition is genetically inherited – and there is still no evidence of this in "schizophrenia" – that would still not imply that pharmaceutical substances would necessarily be the correct treatment. There are many psychological and social approaches that can help the condition on a day-to-day basis.

On the other hand, some conditions might be under-diagnosed by doctors who are determined to believe that all mental health problems are socially rather than genetically influenced. There is much dis-ease that is indeed socially induced: poverty, unemployment, bereavement and many other social conditions are exceedingly distressing and can lead to any number of physical conditions as well as mental instability. The appropriate treatment for these conditions is social. However, this does not mean that *all* physical conditions and states of mental instability are necessarily socially induced. Some people may like to believe that all life's problems emanate from multi-national companies or from fluoridisation of the water supply or from black people or from the influence of the planets or from heaven knows what. Single-issue fanatics – whether they favour genetic or social influences – have answers for everything. When these people become doctors, the end result can be very dangerous. They may see what they believe they see. Their diagnoses will come in clusters, not because particular problems actually exist but because those doctors *believe* that this precise condition is what they are seeing. They cut corners because they believe that standard professional disciplines of observation and consideration are unnecessary. They pronounce the diagnosis (often in Latin) with a sincere look and with nods of the head, and they may nonetheless be *totally* wrong. This may not matter greatly over issues such as food allergies or vitamin and trace element deficiencies, but it matters very greatly when the diagnosis has all the medical and social significance of conditions such as "schizophrenia" or "paranoia". These conditions – preferably simply labelled "psychosis", making no attempt to specify it further – have to be diagnosed accurately and there are very significant penalties for the patient if they are either over-diagnosed or under-diagnosed. The same is true for addictive or compulsive behaviour of any kind. It is vitally important to get an accurate diagnosis.

At the extreme, in totalitarian states, the diagnosis of mental illness is used for political purposes. I do not need to labour the point here other than to say that Hitler and Stalin, and all dictators throughout history and at the present time, have had doctors willing to do their bidding. Simply being a doctor is no guarantee that one has even basic common sense and humanity: it means no more than that one is clever enough to pass particular examinations.

Manic depression or alcoholism

Manic depression is over-diagnosed. We all have some measure of periodic variability of mood state. Just because we go up and down in our moods, sometimes being a long way up and sometimes being a long way down, does not mean that we have manic depression. This is particularly true if we have a high alcohol consumption. Many alcoholics have been misdiagnosed as having manic depression. Needless to say, they themselves are delighted with that diagnosis because it means that there is an acceptable, understandable cause for their variation of mood and that it is nothing to do with their own behaviour. Most importantly, it is nothing to do with their alcohol consumption, so all the nagging that they have received from other people is unjustified and should be replaced with sympathy. The diagnosis of "manic depression" should therefore be made only after excluding the possibility of alcoholism by looking at *why* someone drinks rather than looking at what or how much or when or in what way alcohol is drunk. In particular, people suffering from alcoholism *can* go completely dry but in that state their mood and behaviour become intolerable to other people. The underlying mood disturbance is probably a genetically-inherited defect in neurotransmission systems in the mood centres of the brain. Any mood-altering substance or process will therefore alleviate the sense of inner emptiness that is caused by defects in neurotransmission. Alcohol is only one of those substances. This illustrates the fact that "alcoholism" is really a misnomer: it names the illness after one of its "treatments".

People who have this addictive problem – which I believe should best be termed "neurotransmission disease"-may put down alcohol but will commonly promptly pick up nicotine or sugar or gambling or another mood-altering substance or process in its place. Thus, the diagnosis of "alcoholism" is tricky in itself, even before excluding it when considering the possibility of a diagnosis of "manic depression". Finding the correct diagnosis and giving the correct treatment is therefore exceedingly complex. The worst possible solution to this diagnostic and therapeutic challenge is simply to bang in one medicine after another. Patients deserve better than that.

Personality disorder. Personality inadequacy. Borderline personality

These diagnoses may be little short of insulting to the patients. There is a wide range of "normal" personalities. Extremes should not be pathologised by giving them medical names. Doctors may create a problem – at least in their own minds – simply by labelling it. They may diagnose too readily and interfere too much. Just because a diagnosis may appear in the *International Classification of Diseases* or in *The Diagnostic and Statistical Manual* does not mean necessarily that it actually exists. It means no more than that eminent members of the medical profession currently agree that it does exist as a separate entity. When we look back in history to blood-letting, leaching, cupping and various other barbaric practices agreed upon by eminent members of the medical profession in former years, we should not take it for granted that the days of incorrect diagnosis and treatment by eminent members of the medical profession are now over. In the field of rheumatology in the last ten years, the discovery of a new blood test revealed that the previous standard classification of various diseases was fundamentally wrong. That is not a disaster: it is progress. I hope that exactly the same will happen in the field of psychiatry when more is understood about particular aspects of brain biochemistry.

However, we need not wait for these advances before challenging existing classifications. We have to have good reason to do so and in the case of so-called personality disorder, personality inadequacy or borderline personality there certainly is good reason: patients should be treated with respect and dignity and not be given fanciful diagnoses prior to being drugged as a matter almost of routine by the medical profession in its desire to classify by putting everyone into one box or another. In the field of mental illness I doubt whether many current diagnoses will stand the test of time. Correspondingly, I hope that anti-depressants, tranquillisers and sleeping tablets will not continue to be as popular as they are now. I myself believe that these substances should be avoided altogether. They don't help, they do cause problems in their own right and they are often used in suicides. Most of all, there is no convincing scientific evidence of their efficacy and there is a great deal of justified concern over their use. One wonders at times if some doctors first make the decision to prescribe and then try to find a diagnosis to justify that decision.

"Borderline personality" in simple terms means "nearly mad". Why is it necessary to make this diagnosis at all? One can understand that doctors want to be helpful and that they therefore look to classify in order to be able to treat appropriately. However, this principle falls down catastrophically when the concept of "treatment" is primarily pharmacological. Again, the decision to prescribe a drug may precede consideration of whether it is absolutely necessary to do so and whether the patient will really be helped or hindered by its use and whether there might be some other non-pharmaceutical approach that would be at least as effective if not more so. At times doctors may not be the best people to provide help. We may diagnose and prescribe too much. Other people may have different insights and may be able to provide help in a way that does not risk the side effects – let alone the desecration of the human spirit – of pharmaceutical drugs.

"Anxiety" or "stress"

Anxiety and stress are natural human states that can be protective and even creative. If we are not frightened when under threat, we might miss the opportunity to defend ourselves. Anxiety is not necessarily a handicap in such a situation. Indeed, when we are under threat, we sometimes find very creative ways of protecting ourselves and even reversing the process in a counter-attack. A stressful situation is not necessarily damaging at all: it may concentrate the mind so well that we actually function better when we are under pressure and when the stakes are raised.

Different people may react in different ways when under stress. The same external stressor may cause different internal stress reactions in different people or in the same person at different times. Some people are demolished by a relatively straightforward cause of stress that would be shrugged off by someone else or even used to stimulate creativity. For example, some people react very badly to financial stress whereas others are stimulated by it. Financial brokers thrive on it in a game of wits against each other, and the successful combatants are rewarded with telephone number salaries and bonuses. Lesser mortals could not stand the heat and would have no wish to be in that particular kitchen.

Similarly, acute emergencies bring out the best in some people and the worst in others. We all have our own perceptions of which forms of stress we find acceptable and which are unacceptable. Some people enjoy big dippers on fair grounds and others enjoy rock climbing. Each of us may have a particular activity that gives us a "buzz" from the risk involved. Conversely, probably none of us enjoys a telephone call from a bank manager saying that the overdraft facility has been cancelled. In this way, some risks would be considered to be stimulating whereas others would be very draining.

For a doctor to diagnose "anxiety" or "stress" may therefore be very presumptuous. He or she may simply be observing a human reaction that is completely appropriate in the circumstance involving that particular patient. An appropriate response by the doctor might be "I am not surprised you feel like that. Have you considered various alternative courses of action?". This would leave responsibility in the hands of the patient and he or she might learn from the experience. Writing a prescription to take away the symptoms would, by contrast, give the impression that "anxiety" or "stress" are simply the unfortunate consequences of quirks of fate that have descended upon the hapless patient who had nothing to do with their cause. Under such circumstances the prescription of a drug would do nothing to help patients to change their behaviour or their relationships or circumstances or whatever it was that was leading to the stress symptoms in the first place. Further, they would be prevented from learning from the experience and, even further, they would be likely to become emotionally dependent upon the drug, believing that they needed it in order to suppress uncomfortable feelings. By contrast, the most beneficial "prescription" may be a recommendation to consider a change in lifestyle or in personal and professional circumstances. The last thing that patients need when they are in challenging personal or social situations is a retreat into the unreality of a drug-induced haze. When doctors say that they are prescribing a drug in order to help patients to have a clear mind, they are in fact achieving the exact opposite: their patients are not being encouraged to face up to their difficulties and to recognise their own contributions to them.

When patients externalise their problems, as if there is no connection between their behaviour and their feelings, it makes those problems *less* accessible to change. These patients may view themselves as being powerless over their disturbed feelings and over the events that lead to them. The true situation is that we feel anxious or stressed particularly when our behaviour does not match our values. If we do something that we know is wrong then we will feel bad about it. In such circumstances we have the choice of either changing our behaviour or changing our values. From the moment we take a tablet, we reduce the possibility of seeing our own involvement in the circumstances that led to our disturbed feelings. Even when we are in stressful or dangerous circumstances that were not of our own choosing, we may sometimes with profit ask ourselves how we came to be in those situations in the first place. Responsible doctors, in my view, should primarily help patients to examine their values, behaviour and relationships so that "anxiety" or "stress" is minimised. These symptoms are not mysterious in any way: they are directly associated with each patient's personal philosophy. Prescribing medications results in a disconnection in the patient's mind between cause and effect and, far from being helpful, that is very disruptive.

"Depression" versus "sadness"

Sadness is the normal human response to distressing events. It should be treated solely with understanding, support from family and friends, and time. It does not require treatment with medication, which can in fact be harmful by getting in the way of the natural emotional and social healing processes.

"Sadness" should be differentiated from "depression" because when a doctor diagnoses "depression", this may sometimes lead almost automatically to a prescription for an "anti-depressant". If the true diagnosis is "sadness" then both the diagnosis of "depression" and the prescription for an "anti-depressant" may be too hasty.

Unfortunately doctors do not give up the habit of prescribing without fighting a rearguard action. They tend to create new diagnostic categories in order to establish their right to prescribe. After all, they might feel singularly naked if deprived of their prescription pads: they might not know what else to do if they cannot write a prescription. Consequently the term "clinical depression" has recently come into vogue so that doctors can emphasise that the word "clinical" means that the patient really needs to be under medical care and that he or she has much more than a simple emotional or social problem. The new diagnosis re-establishes the right to prescribe an anti-depressant.

By the same token, the diagnosis of "agitated depression" enshrines the right of the doctor to prescribe both a tranquilliser and an anti-depressant. Similarly the term "psychotic depression" means that the doctor intends to prescribe an anti-depressant as well as an anti-psychotic medication.

There are no diagnostic tests that are capable of confirming any of these diagnoses. They are simply points of view and, as such, they are fallible rather than cast in stone.

Prescribing drugs is always the easy way out for a doctor on three counts. Firstly it establishes that the doctor is in charge. Secondly it demonstrates that "something has been done" – which can be a useful piece of evidence in court or to the General Medical Council if the patient commits suicide or if something else goes dreadfully wrong. Thirdly, the patient may be very grateful to have a "real" diagnosis rather than have to face up to the need to re-examine his or her own philosophy and lifestyle.

By contrast, in my view, the most responsible approach is to provide a dignified and secure environment for the patient – either on an out-patient or in-patient basis – and reduce medications to a minimum or even cut them out altogether so that the doctor can see how the patient behaves in a supportive environment and when not drugged out of his or her mind with one substance or another.

The practical problem with this approach comes from trying to provide a dignified and supportive environment within a publicly-funded facility. When demands are high and motivation is low, it is easier for all concerned simply to bang in another drug and justify it with a diagnosis that sounds important. In earlier years, Largactil (Chlorpromazine) was referred to as "a liquid cosh" because of the tranquillising – some would say stupefying – effect that it had on "difficult" patients. Its side effect of jaundice was seen as troublesome, but the principle of "knocking out" a patient was rarely challenged. Nowadays more sophisticated drugs may be used, but the principle behind their prescription remains much the same.

Depression and addiction

Depression may in fact be "untreated" addictive disease. People who are addicts have an inner sense of emptiness, which may be due to a genetically-inherited defect in neurotransmission in the mood centres of the brain. They feel "depressed" for no accountable reason. Long before they took drugs or drank alcohol or got involved with eating disorders or other addictive or compulsive behaviours, they will have felt this inner sense of emptiness or loneliness even when surrounded by friends or family and even when their lives may have been relatively free from obvious problems. Depending upon the social circumstances of their families, some will be rich and others poor, some will come from broken homes and others from stable homes, some may have suffered abuse or abandonment and others not, but all will have a sense of isolation. Viewed in this light, their subsequent addictive behaviour becomes fully explicable: they will try to change the way they feel. They do not drink alcohol, use drugs, binge or starve, gamble or do other addictive and compulsive things merely as a result of peer pressure or experiment, but because they discover that these things produce an almost magical mood-altering effect: they make them feel better about themselves when nothing else in life has had the capacity to do that. Obviously, once they have discovered a substance or process that works in this way, they will be unlikely ever to give it up voluntarily. They only do so when the pain of continuing to use it becomes greater than the perceived pain of giving it up. In that ultimate dilemma many addicts commit suicide. The Samaritans estimate that 40% of all suicides are among alcoholics alone. When one adds in those suicides that occur in people who have problems with drug addiction or eating disorders, compulsive gambling and other forms of addictive behaviour, it is clear that the majority of suicides are found among people who have an addictive tendency.

It is therefore tautologous to think in terms of "dual diagnosis" of addiction and depression. Other than in physiological circumstances – such as after childbirth when a depressive state may be a natural response – depression is the cardinal sign of addictive disease. Depression and addiction – or, at least, an addictive tendency – are the same thing.

It follows that anything that "treats" depression will itself have a potential for addiction. For example, alcohol is a treatment for depression. So is cannabis or cocaine or heroin or sugar or caffeine or gambling or work or exercise or shopping and spending or any other substance or process that is mood-altering. They are all the "wrong" treatments for depression because they all have damaging side-effects in the long term. This same caveat applies to mood-altering prescription drugs such as tranquillisers, anti-depressants and sleeping tablets. The very fact that they have the capacity to alter the mood means that they are addictive to people who have addictive disease. They tend not to be seen in this light because they are usually slow to act and subsequently slow to reveal withdrawal effects after their use has been discontinued. Nonetheless they are addictive to people with addictive disease, and this can be seen by what happens to those people when the mood-altering prescription drugs are stopped: they revert to the original depressive state and they commonly try to "treat" that by resorting to other addictive substances and processes. They come out of one addiction and go into another.

It has been argued that the correct treatment would therefore be to maintain the patients on mood-altering pharmaceutical substances for life. This is a policy of despair. Mood-altering prescription drugs provide a very restricted emotional life, with neither the highs nor the lows that bring colour to an otherwise drab existence. People who take mood-altering prescription medications on a continuing basis become very restricted in their capacity to gain any value from life other than in purely economic terms or in terms of physical survival. Their spirits are dead. Often they despair and commit suicide, using the very drugs that were prescribed to "*treat*" them.

This tragedy can be avoided by guiding them towards the Twelve Step programme of the Anonymous Fellowships. This is far more than a blueprint for a happy life: it is the vital treatment for addictive disease itself. The essential therapeutic paradox of this treatment is that when one addict reaches out to help another anonymously, it is the first one – the giver – who feels better. The recipient may also do so, but the giver, in taking his or her mind off self and putting it on to the other addict, receives a burst of neuro-chemicals leading to mood-alteration that is the equivalent of the effects of any of the addictive substances or processes that were previously used.

The immense advantages of this non-medicinal treatment are that it is self-induced and dose-responsive. In other words, it is not dependent upon other people doing anything at all and it can be used at any time and in any place according to need. The further advantage is that it has no damaging side effects. It is a lovely thing to do, anyway. Its only disadvantage is that, like other "treatments" for depression, its effects wear off in time so that it has to be repeated. Thus, attendance at meetings of the Anonymous Fellowships and working the Twelve Step programme is a treatment that has to be continued for life. It is the straight alternative to using other mood-altering substances or processes. People who use alcohol as their particular "treatment" may not want to go to Alcoholics Anonymous and work its Twelve Step programme but it is a straight choice between that behaviour and continuing to drink alcohol with all its damaging side-effects. The same principle applies to all other mood-altering substances and processes: the straight choice is between continuing their use or working the Twelve Step programme of an appropriate Anonymous Fellowship. Depression, when seen in this light, can be treated effectively on a continuing basis without the use of any pharmaceutical substance. Emotions Anonymous exists for those people who have never tried to "treat" their depression with specific mood-altering substances or processes.

The catch in understanding addictive disease is that it affects not only the mood but also the perception mechanisms of the mind. The disease "tells" the sufferer that he or she has not got it. This has devastating consequences. After all, why should one seek treatment for an illness that one has not got? The basic psychopathology of addictive disease is denial. This is countered by attendance at meetings of appropriate Anonymous Fellowships. One may not be able to see oneself but one can see other people and then, on discovering that their stories have an uncanny resemblance to one's own, one begins to recognise that one must therefore have the same problem.

"Alcoholism", "addiction", "eating disorders"

There are significant dangers in under-diagnosing these conditions, particularly in the early stages of the illness. Many major illnesses have the inner emptiness of addictive disease (self-treated with nicotine, alcohol, drugs or sugar) as an important precursor. Early diagnosis and appropriate treatment of addictive disease will often be life-saving. Correspondingly, there are significant dangers in over-diagnosis: adolescent problems, habituation, cultural norms or stupidity can all be misdiagnosed as addiction. The Shorter PROMIS Questionnaire (which can be found on www.promis.co.uk) specifically differentiates addictive tendencies from each other and from non-addictive behaviour.

Many people drink alcohol as part of their cultural norm. For example, if we were to sweep the streets at night for people who were drunk we might pick up a fair number of students, journalists, soldiers or coal miners. This does not mean that they are alcoholic: it simply means that they come from a culture which tends at times to be heavy drinking. Similarly, finding traces of cannabis in the bedroom of a teenager does not mean that he or she is an addict, even though cannabis is a major addictive drug. It may simply mean that he or she is doing what others of his or her generation often do in experimenting with mood-altering substances or processes. Discovering that a young girl has been self-inducing vomiting does not mean that she is bulimic. Many young girls indulge in this behaviour when they are under stress. Only a few of them turn out in due course to have full-blown bulimia nervosa, just as only a few of the people who are on diets turn out to have anorexia and only a few of the drunken students turn out to be alcoholic. The crucial differentiation is not what someone does, or how much or how little, or when or in what circumstances, but *why*. All the questions in the Shorter PROMIS Questionnaire target the "*why*" of addictive behaviour. This is not something that changes over the years or in different circumstances and it therefore makes no difference whether the behaviour is past or present. If one has *ever* had the addictive behaviour outlined in the Shorter PROMIS Questionnaire, then it can easily break out again. The fact is that people who have addictive disease can – and often do – put down addictive substances and processes for a time. However, they do so at a dreadful cost to their mood and behaviour. They may become angry and resentful and make life extremely difficult for other people. This condition is generally termed the "dry drunk" state even in the case of addictive substances or processes that have no connection with alcohol. In fact the "dry drunk" state illustrates addictive disease in its purest form – before the recourse to "treatment" with various mood-altering substances or processes. It reveals precisely what it is that the sufferers from addictive disease are trying to treat: the inner emptiness and despair, anger and resentment, blame and self-pity that are the fundamental characteristics of their mood disorder.

Chemical Damage

As already mentioned, over forty million prescriptions for anti-depressants, tranquillisers or sleeping tablets are written each year in the U.K. An increasing number of children, even those in their pre-teen years, are prescribed Prozac and other drugs for "depression" and Ritalin (an amphetamine derivative) for "attention-deficient hyperactivity disorder". These diagnoses have been placed in inverted commas quite deliberately because it is questionable whether either exists, particularly in young children. My own book, *Preventing Addiction*, (PROMIS 2000) is targeted towards exactly this age group. I believe that many of the behavioural disturbances seen in young children are in fact the precursors of addiction. Far from prescribing for these children, we should give them an understanding of addictive disease and we should help them to become familiar with the basic principles of a Twelve Step programme. Anything is preferable to a pharmacological assault upon the delicate developing tissues of the child's brain. Our knowledge of brain biochemistry is still in its infancy and the powers of the brain to put itself right are as remarkable as those of other parts of the body. Doctors should be discouraged from prescribing any mood-altering chemical to adults, let alone to children, until they have demonstrated that there is no other effective clinical approach. The Twelve Step programme should be the first, rather than the last, clinical approach that is tried.

Psychological Damage

"The sick state" may be falsely diagnosed. Patients may sometimes be incapacitated or damaged by seeing themselves in this light. When they perceive themselves as being ill or incapacitated, their minds may become preoccupied by that condition and they may become less able to function effectively in their normal daily lives. For this reason, doctors and psychologists, therapists or counsellors, should never diagnose a patient as being "sick" or "ill" or having a "disease" or even "dis-ease" unless they can substantiate their diagnosis as far as it is possible to do so.

Just as doctors may over-diagnose medical conditions, so psychologists, therapists, psychotherapists and counsellors may over-diagnose psychological conditions. Patients may be led towards believing that they have particular taints from childhood or particular propensities towards one form of behaviour or another. For example, saying that someone was abused or abandoned in childhood might overlook the fact that we all have difficult or even abusive childhoods to some degree – although this does not diminish the significance of extreme experience. Similarly, saying that someone is "co-dependent" (in my view a very confusing term because it has so many different interpretations) may lead him or her to assume all sorts of self-limiting psychological traits.

The pathologising of childhood experience may be unfair to parents or other carers and may be counter-productive for the individual by leading him or her to become obsessed with childhood events and their damaging influence rather than focusing upon the adult capacity to surmount childhood trauma and move on. The belief of analytical psychotherapists that much of our future psychological life is determined by early childhood experience is manifestly wrong. Childhood experiences are important but they can be surmounted at any time. New experiences can override the effects of old. *Aging Well* by George Vaillant (Little, Brown 2002) gives an account of people who have been studied for over fifty years since they were recruited as teenagers in the Study of Adult Development at Harvard University. It contains (page 5) the following observations:

"As they surmount the inevitable crises of aging, the study members seem constantly to be reinventing their lives. They surprise us even as they surprise themselves. In moments of sorrow, loss and defeat, many still convince us that they find their lives eminently worthwhile. They do not flinch from acknowledging how hard life is, but they also never lose sight of why one might want to keep on living it."

If these people can "re-invent" their lives when they are nearing the end, this is surely good evidence of their capacity to do so throughout their lives.

Strangely, the psycho-dynamic belief in the Oedipus Complex, first formulated by Sigmund Freud, points to children sexualising their relationship with parents. It would appear that Sigmund Freud, Melanie Klein and the rest of her breed lay the responsibility for childhood sexual abuse, which is distressingly common with estimates of 25% or more, on the children themselves! Strange indeed that the genuine pathology of sexual abuse should be blamed on the child while the fiction of early childhood permanent conditioning (unless treated with lengthy expensive analysis) should be perpetuated. In any case, Melanie Klein's abandonment of her own children is hardly a recommendation for her ideas.

Even so, deeply stressful experiences at any age can become locked into the psyche and form the focus of post-traumatic stress disorder. This should be treated straightforwardly through Eye Movement Desensitisation and Reprocessing (EMDR). Lesser traumas should be understood as simply part of life's experience from which we can learn and grow, rather than as something that has damaged us for ever. It can even become counter-productive to review childhood experiences in such depth that the end result is that the patient becomes an emotional cripple, obsessed with complexes of one kind or another, rather than someone who is free to get on with life without focusing upon every possible psychological nuance.

Blame and self-pity are usually unhealthy and unproductive whereas acceptance and gratitude are usually healthy and creative. Too much psychotherapy can be a very bad thing if the end result is a closed, suspicious and self-obsessed personality rather than one that is open and free.

Helping people towards the healthy state of spontaneity, creativity and enthusiasm should be the primary goal of all therapeutic interventions. Any therapeutic intervention that leaves an individual believing that he or she is permanently scarred, and without the chance of healing, is therefore very damaging. Exactly this accusation is sometimes laid at the door of those who diagnose addictive disease and who recommend a Twelve Step approach that emphasises the individual's powerlessness over it. In this special case, however, the process of surrender and admitting defeat (in the battle to prove that one can use mood-altering substances or processes without ill effect as other people often can) is the very process that provides the power to get on with life, unburdened by the recurrent calamities of active addiction. People who have an addictive tendency are initially very reluctant to accept this powerlessness in themselves although they may recognise it in other people. The most fervent opponents of the diagnosis of addictive disease and the Twelve Step treatment programme are therefore very often people who have addictive tendencies themselves. This does not mean that those of us who espouse Twelve Step treatment programmes for addictive disease can ride roughshod over all scientific principles of diagnostic and therapeutic thoroughness. However, it does mean that those who attack us might benefit from first examining their own behaviour – just as we ourselves have had to do.

Communication Failure.

As mentioned previously, the process of communication should be judged by what arrives in the patient's mind rather than by what was said by the doctor. The doctor may say something perfectly clearly, but if it did not arrive in the patient's mind, then it has not been communicated. Nurse practitioners, counsellors and other staff may be called in to use their special communicative skills to help patients to be more relaxed and hence gain greater understanding of their clinical conditions and what needs to be done for them.

Medical practice has a wide variation in the demands for communication skills. A laboratory scientist or full-time academic researcher might have little need for the skill of putting patients at ease. By contrast, a general medical practitioner might find it very difficult to function at all without that skill. This is important because those general practitioners who find themselves in the "wrong slot" in this respect might be tempted to reach for a prescription pad at the first available opportunity rather than to listen to their patients, discuss things with them and provide them with comfort and support. As a general principle, doctors who lack natural communicative skills should be encouraged to find an area of clinical practice where there is little or no contact with live patients. There are many ways of helping people without necessarily having direct contact with them.

It is questionable whether communication skills as such can ever be taught. Some improvement in natural ability may be possible through training, but ultimately, as in all areas of life, it might be best simply to accept, when confronted with the evidence, that one lacks a particular skill. In this respect I write from the experience of having tried for fifteen years to prove that I could be a professional musician: I could not – I was not good enough and I lacked the basic gifts that professional musicians require. Accepting that fact did not diminish me: it helped me to re-focus my attention on activities in which I did have more natural talent. On that same principle, there should be no disgrace when doctors accept that their talents lead them in one direction rather than another. The tragedy for patients, as far as general practice is concerned, is that doctors sometimes come into this discipline as a result of failing in others. A mismatch in this respect can result in a very dispirited doctor and a series of damaged patients over the course of an entire professional lifetime. That whole process could have been avoided if it had been accepted that communication skills, like musicianship, are special gifts that are not given to all of us in equal measure. Patients – and audiences – deserve the best of us.

Chapter Five

Philosophical Complacency

"The NHS is under-funded and poorly administered"

Doctors and patients may not understand that an effective health service can in fact be provided on *any* budget, provided that there is clear definition of what is to be *excluded*. Otherwise health services become a bottomless pit of expectations exceeding resource. That inevitably leads to dissatisfaction and resentment in both doctors and patients. The perpetual complaint that the NHS is under-funded and poorly administered may result in doctors and patients focusing upon justifying what they *cannot* do rather than on seeing what they *can* do. This is obviously counterproductive.

It may be true that the NHS is relatively under-funded in comparison with the health services of other countries. It may also be true that services in one part of the UK may be relatively under-funded in comparison with those in another. It may also be true that some clinical disciplines are relatively under-funded in comparison with others or that they are under-funded for the expectations put upon them by Government or health authorities. Even so, the fact remains that, in any area of life whatever, one *can* deliver a service according to one's budget. The fact that one may want more – or deserve more – should not detract from focusing upon what one *can* achieve.

In medical terms a doctor or other healthcare provider has to think of what is appropriate for an individual or community to receive within a defined budget. For example, an old person would obviously benefit very considerably from a cataract operation. This is inexpensive in itself, it adds dramatically to the quality of life and it is also a sensible precautionary measure in reducing the incidence of falls leading to fractures. By contrast that same patient's cancer might not necessarily benefit from treatment. It might be slow growing, and treatment might not necessarily add either to the quality or length of life. Just because something *could* be done does not necessarily mean that it *should*.

Similarly, when considering the population at large, it might be possible to reduce the incidence of cancer of the breast if one were to get all surgeons to focus upon this clinical condition and nothing else. Cancer of the breast is indeed an extremely distressing condition that is well deserving of our support. For this to be done at the expense of every other clinical condition – such as cancers of other parts of the body – is obviously not justifiable. Those who suffer from cancer of the breast or those who campaign on their behalf will inevitably believe that the services given to them are under-funded and possibly poorly administered as well. However, these claims have to be seen alongside other competing claims for finite resources. We do not live in a Utopian world but one in which resources are inevitably finite. Resources therefore have to be apportioned with consideration to cost and benefit. To do otherwise is to squander them.

These considerations concerning rationing and apportioning are emotive issues when applied to healthcare – but the importance of healthcare is all the more reason why we should approach these subjects rationally rather than emotively. Doctors should lead the way in this respect.

"The NHS is the envy of the world."

Doctors who believe that the NHS is the envy of the world may close their minds and fail to look at alternatives that might improve patient care. They become so mesmerised with political issues that they may fail to see what is actually happening to patients in clinical terms. Paradoxically, as the service progressively fails, these doctors may defend it even more vigorously. Similarly, patients may cling to it even more desperately in the uninformed fear that there is no viable alternative.

Patients living in a welfare state may make progressively less provision for their own health and welfare because they believe that the State will always provide for them. Further, they may believe that they have rights rather than responsibilities for themselves or for other people. This dependency and entitlement culture leads to further fear and resentment when the service inevitably fails to live up to impossible Utopian goals. The pressure upon doctors to deliver a service that they simply cannot deliver within the resources available may result in doctors becoming very dispirited – and thereby becoming the apex of a whole pyramid of suffering. Party political slogans such as "the NHS is the envy of the world" can be very destructive to all who work within the system – because they cannot meet the expectations of the patients and therefore they know that patients must either change their expectations of the NHS or seek help elsewhere. The belief that "the NHS is the envy of the world" is equally destructive to patients when they fail to make proper provision for the health and welfare of their own families and for themselves. Politicians – and the doctors who follow them – should watch their mouths.

"The Government ought to do something"

When doctors believe this to such an extent that they become disempowered in their own work, failing to achieve the best of their own potential within the resources available, they may progressively fail to see that they themselves are becoming mere tools of the state rather than independent thinkers or innovators. They would benefit from asking themselves the question "What could I myself do, irrespective of what the Government should or should not do?". We are lost from the moment that we delegate all responsibility to Government.

Patients who believe that "the Government ought to do something" may become stuck in a dependency culture and do progressively less to help themselves. Instead of spending their money on health and welfare and education – aspects of life that have the potential to bring considerable benefit to themselves and their families – they may fritter it away on trivia. The Registrar-General's abstract of statistics now shows that the average family spends more on cigarettes, alcohol and gambling than they do on housing, let alone on their own health and welfare. The Welfare State may have reduced some problems – although general improvements in housing and sanitation have probably been a greater influence – but it has certainly created others. A society that fritters its life away while expecting the Government to look after issues that really matter – such as health and education – is a very sick society. Perhaps the process should be reversed: the Government should focus upon the trivial aspects of life while individuals should be encouraged to take more responsibility for themselves in the really important ones. Obviously neither extreme is immediately practicable – but the challenge has to be made in order to demonstrate that total reliance upon Government is just as dangerous, if not more so, as providing no Government service at all.

A further factor is that society may become less caring on the assumption that the Government will always provide for those who are least capable of helping themselves. The Welfare State in this respect can become the cause of a great deal of suffering. People who might otherwise have helped their friends and neighbours might retreat into saying "The Government ought to do something". When presented with evidence that it does not, they might respond that it *should* - do so rather than by seeing what they could do to help others. Thus the Welfare State can be the cause of the Inverse Care Law, first coined by the communist GP Dr Julian Tudor-Hart, which states that those most in need of help are least likely to get it.

"The Government knows best."

Many doctors work in the Department of Health or in other administrative positions within the health and welfare services. When they believe that they themselves know best, they may be right or they may be catastrophically wrong.

An example of where the Government probably does know best is in the subject of epidemiology, the study of infections and other illnesses within communities. However, even in this field there has been some anxiety about whether the Government really does always know best. I am not an epidemiologist and I therefore have to acknowledge the limit of my understanding. That being said, however, the Government has so far been totally wrong in its predictions of an epidemic of AIDS in British-born heterosexuals. Evidence from the sheer number of illegitimate pregnancies still occurring today shows that many people have not changed their behaviour concerning unprotected sexual intercourse. Yet still there is no roaring epidemic of AIDS.

There is evidence that many homosexuals have changed their behaviour towards having "safe sex" but even this change of behaviour is far from universal. There are limits to what the Government can achieve positively in a totalitarian state, let alone in a democracy such as ours. By contrast, Government policies can at times be extremely damaging. As mentioned previously, the policy of Methadone maintenance in the treatment of heroin addiction is an unmitigated disaster. Methadone is an oral substitute for injectable heroin and is a major addictive substance in its own right. Thus, treating heroin addicts with Methadone does not treat their addiction at all – it simply transfers it from one substance to another. In the UK more than a million prescriptions for Methadone are now written every year. This is scandalous evidence of lack of care for the addicts themselves. They could be helped towards total abstinence through working the Twelve Step programme of Narcotics Anonymous but instead they are simply written off as being hopeless, stupid, depraved or even undeserving. The purpose of Methadone maintenance programmes is not to help the addicts themselves but to try to prevent AIDS and hepatitis B and C from getting into the heterosexual population via needle-using addicted prostitutes. Thus, one sector of the community is written off while trying to protect another. This is not only bad clinical practice, it is also unethical, particularly when alternative methods of treatment can achieve total abstinence. In this respect the Government most certainly does *not* know best: it is fundamentally wrong.

Another legitimate concern over the concept that "the Government knows best" is that doctors who work in Government departments may lose sight of the clinical realities of those of us who work daily with patients. They may produce recommendations and protocols and even commands that are designed to have the patients' best interests at heart, but these may nonetheless produce the opposite of what was intended, because of practical difficulties in delivering the service to each and every patient. A recent example was the recommendation that in times of epidemics of respiratory infections, such as influenza, each GP should visit all the elderly people on his or her list every day. In some medical practices this would amount to hundreds of visits to these vulnerable patients. The theory, formulated in an ivory tower, looks wonderful; practical implementation would be impossible. Doctors in clinical practice may at times, such as in this example, feel that they have become hounded and, as a result, they may do very bad work indeed. The Government may have had good intentions but they pave the way to hell.

The sheer arrogance of Government departments can be dumbfounding, as when they announce that they have had consultations with the public when in fact all they have done is to publish their own proposals on a website and then put in their own jobsworths to fend off any comments or suggestions that may challenge their own predetermined policy. "Representative democracy" does not describe this process very well. In this respect, Government departments are little short of totalitarian in their instincts. Yet even then it might never occur to them that "the Government knows best" is anything less than the absolute truth.

"The private sector will always be better"

When people say this, they are blind to the truth and one might question their motives. The private sector can be just as incompetent as the state sector and there is sometimes little to choose between the avarice of the private sector and the arrogance of the state sector. Sometimes, as in the occasional case of cosmetic surgery, patients may actually be damaged by getting what they pay for.

The majority of doctors working in the private sector will be just as responsible and caring as their colleagues in the state sector. The universality of the assumption that the private sector will always deliver a better service is nevertheless questionable. There are considerable advantages for private doctors in their capacity to choose the facilities, equipment, staff and services available to them – but this does not mean that their choices are always sensible or necessarily primarily for the benefit of their patients. There are proportionately as many charlatans and dishonest doctors in the private sector as there are in the state sector. Periodically doctors get caught defrauding the NHS, but equally doctors get caught defrauding insurance companies. They may not get caught ripping off their patients – and some patients are incredibly gullible in this respect – but dishonesty, or at least disingenuousness, certainly exists and it is probably commonplace.

Private doctors are fond of saying that they like to give time to their patients in order to practise "good" medicine and they blame the Government for not training more doctors. Also they may believe that the Government should offer a "choice" of services. These beliefs are entirely self-motivated: the only real beneficiaries would be private doctors themselves. The challenge that can legitimately be laid at the door of the private sector is to ask how it would cater for the *entire* population and how it would fund the training of doctors, nurses and other staff as well as research programmes and preventive measures.

Private hospitals and medical insurance companies tend to ignore this challenge. The majority of their claims are for routine procedures, consultations and minor operations. Indeed, most medical insurers do not even cover chronic illnesses. This is a standard policy exclusion. There are no Accident and Emergency facilities in the private sector. Few private hospitals have high dependency units. Nor do they generally have intensive care departments of the standard found in the NHS. There are minimal private training facilities for doctors or nurses; instead the private sector is content to siphon away the top end of the skill in medical professionals. The private sector, and particularly medical insurance companies, should be more open and honest in this respect. They should cut out all pretence of "assisting" the state sector and recognise that they are parasitic upon it when they cream off the best people and the easy aspects of the work.

This does not mean that there is no place for a private sector or even that it could never replace a state-funded system altogether. However, it does mean that the private sector should put its own house in order before criticising the state sector. Doctors in both private and state sectors should beware of pontificating on the superiority of either system.

A state system may wish to limit medical costs – but so do private medical insurance companies and health maintenance organisations. A state system may wish to provide care for those most in need but they are heavily dependent in this respect upon the services provided through private charities. Neither system has all the virtues or all the vices.

One thing that can be said, particularly after reading *The Public/Private Mix for Health*, edited by Alan Maynard and Gordon McLaghlan (Nuffield Provincial Hospitals Trust 1982), is that doctors will turn any system anywhere in the world to their own advantage. There are of course notable individual exceptions but, in general, doctors in state systems will tend to follow the principle of any trade union in demanding more pay for less work. Conversely, doctors in the private sector will follow the example of city slickers and make a fast buck wherever they can, putting up their fees particularly when an insurance company is footing the bill.

As I see it, the best system will be one where patients take responsibility for their own healthcare maintenance – with charitable support for specific clinical conditions where this is impossible – and doctors go out of business if they fail to provide a service that is helpful to their patients and appreciated by them. It has always worried me that the concept of medical practice being part of the general marketplace should be viewed with scorn. Why should doctors *not* compete with each other? Why should they *not* go out of business if they fail to provide services of an adequate standard or those that are valued by their patients? Why should they *not* make profits from the sick? The failure to make a profit means that they are not providing a service that is valued either by the individual patients or by a charity or by the Government, depending upon who pays the bill. The failure to focus upon the sick, rather than the worried well, would lead one to question why they became doctors in the first place.

There should be no nostalgia, remembering the "good old days" of paternalistic medical practice. Doctors should compete with each other and the provision of personal care to patients should be the subject of their competition. Patients should not simply be treated on a production line as "interesting cases". They have their own perspectives and values and they have every right to expect doctors to consider them. The one advantage of the private sector in this respect is that ultimately the patients hold the whip hand. They get the service that they value or they go elsewhere – and so they should.

Other books in the series

Preventing Addiction

Cigarette Smoking. Fifteen reasons for continuing to smoke (or not)

Healing

Common Sense in the Treatment of Eating Disorders

Spiritual Awakening. Working the Twelve Step programme

Inside the Madness

How to Combat Alcoholism and Addiction

How to Combat Anorexia, Bulimia and Compulsive Overeating

Spirituality for Atheists and Agnostics

A New Life. Healing depression

Compulsive Helping

Healthy Relationships

Prescription Drug Addiction. My doctor gave it to me

Behavioural Addictions: Workaholism. Shopaholism. Exercise Addiction. Gambling and Risk Taking. Self-Harming. Obsessive Compulsive Disorder

False Medical Gods

Detoxification and Harm Minimisation

Childhood Abuse and Abandonment

Healing Emotional Trauma with E.M.D.R.

Healing Emotional Trauma with Psychodrama

Treating Chronic Relapse. Not again

Help: The Dairy of a Private Doctor

- **Vol 1: I will *not* make do.** The philosophy and politics of help
- **Vol 2: Daughters are Difficult.** Professional help in clinical practice
- **Vol 3: Henry is a Good Man.** The boundaries of help
- **Vol 4: Robin's turn.** Beyond help

dangerous doctors